## WHAT MAKES THE RICE DIET SOLUTION THE ULTIMATE ANSWER TO ALL YOUR DIET NEEDS?

**SOLID TRACK RECORD**: Turning out success stories since 1939, the Rice Diet Program is the original, most effective diet to use nutrition to achieve not only safe and rapid weight loss but also the prevention and reversal of chronic disease.

**RAPID WEIGHT LOSS**: The average "Ricer" loses up to thirty pounds in the first month!

**LONG-TERM SUCCESS**: Sixty-three percent of people who have lost weight on the Rice Diet report weighing the same or less one year later.

**MEDICALLY SOUND**: The Rice Diet Program is run by Duke University–trained doctors with more than thirty years of medical experience using diet as the primary treatment for long-term weight loss and disease reversal.

**SCIENTIFICALLY PROVEN**: Numerous scientific publications, including the *American Journal of Medicine*, have documented the diet's dramatic effects on such life-threatening illnesses as congestive heart failure and heart disease and its risk factors: diabetes, high cholesterol, high blood pressure, and obesity.

**HOLISTIC APPROACH**: The Rice Diet Solution helps you examine root causes of your particular health issues and empowers you to create the life you really desire.

*Ten percent of the net sales of this book
will be donated to educational and charitable causes
that promote health and healing.*

ALSO BY KITTY GURKIN ROSATI

Heal Your Heart:
The New Rice Diet Program for Reversing Heart Disease
Through Nutrition, Exercise, and Spiritual Renewal

# THE
# RICE
# DIET
# SOLUTION

*The World-Famous Low-Sodium, Good-Carb, Detox Diet for Quick and Lasting Weight Loss*

KITTY GURKIN ROSATI,
M.S., R.D., L.D.N., AND
ROBERT ROSATI, M.D.

BERKLEY BOOKS, NEW YORK

**THE BERKLEY PUBLISHING GROUP**
**Published by the Penguin Group**
**Penguin Group (USA) Inc.**
**375 Hudson Street, New York, New York 10014, USA**
Penguin Group (Canada), 90 Eglinton Avenue East, Suite 700, Toronto, Ontario M4P 2Y3, Canada
(a division of Pearson Penguin Canada Inc.)
Penguin Books Ltd., 80 Strand, London WC2R 0RL, England
Penguin Group Ireland, 25 St. Stephen's Green, Dublin 2, Ireland (a division of Penguin Books Ltd.)
Penguin Group (Australia), 250 Camberwell Road, Camberwell, Victoria 3124, Australia
(a division of Pearson Australia Group Pty. Ltd.)
Penguin Books India Pvt. Ltd., 11 Community Centre, Panchsheel Park, New Delhi—110 017, India
Penguin Group (NZ), Cnr. Airborne and Rosedale Roads, Albany, Auckland 1310, New Zealand
(a division of Pearson New Zealand Ltd.)
Penguin Books (South Africa) (Pty.) Ltd., 24 Sturdee Avenue, Rosebank, Johannesburg 2196,
South Africa

Penguin Books Ltd., Registered Offices: 80 Strand, London WC2R 0RL, England

PUBLISHER'S NOTE: Every effort has been made to ensure that the information contained in this book is complete and accurate. However, neither the publisher nor the author is engaged in rendering professional advice or services to the individual reader. The ideas, procedures, and suggestions contained in this book are not intended as a substitute for consulting with your physician. All matters regarding your health require medical supervision. Neither the author nor the publisher shall be liable or responsible for any loss or damage allegedly arising from any information or suggestion in this book.

The recipes contained in this book are to be followed exactly as written. The publisher is not responsible for your specific health or allergy needs that may require medical supervision. The publisher is not responsible for any adverse reactions to the recipes contained in this book. The publisher does not have any control over and does not assume any responsibility for author or third-party websites or their content.

THE RICE DIET SOLUTION

PRINTING HISTORY
Simon & Schuster hardcover edition / 2005
Berkley trade paperback edition / January 2007

Berkley trade paperback ISBN: 978-0-425-21466-4

An application to register this book for cataloging has been submitted to the Library of Congress.

PRINTED IN THE UNITED STATES OF AMERICA

10  9  8  7  6  5  4  3  2  1

*This book is dedicated to all of those who are committed to maximizing their life, to actualizing their gifts, and to passing this passion for healing on to others. Specifically, this includes Dr. Walter Kempner, Dr. Eugene Stead, Rev. Tommy Tyson and his Aqueduct Retreat Center family, my mom (Pat aka Grammy), and our precious son, Chess.*

# CONTENTS

# CHAPTER FOUR

# CHAPTER FIVE

# CHAPTER SIX

# CHAPTER SEVEN

# CHAPTER EIGHT

# CHAPTER NINE

# THE
# RICE
# DIET
# SOLUTION

# PHYSICIAN'S WARNING

Before starting any new diet or exercise program, you should check with your personal physician. This is particularly important if you are taking medications. While on the diet, you should experience a sense of well-being. Indeed, most patients say they haven't felt as well in years. If you don't feel well (particularly if you experience nausea or dizziness on standing), check in with your doctor immediately.

You should be under the supervision of your personal physician if you are taking medications for diabetes, high blood pressure, or congestive heart failure. If you are being treated for diabetes, you will have to have your medications adjusted by your physician as you lose weight. You should not combine the diet with diuretics or medications containing diuretics, but, again, you should not discontinue any medications without your physician's approval. If you are taking lithium or the blood thinner warfarin (coumadin), your physician may have to adjust the dose.

The Rice Diet should not be undertaken by patients who have had resection of part or all of their colon, patients who have had ureteral diversion procedures, or patients with impaired kidney function.

# INTRODUCTION

*It is wonderful, if we chose the right diet, what an extraordinarily small quantity would suffice.*

—Mahatma Gandhi

A re you frustrated with your war on weight? Have you tried any number of diets, lost weight, and then, in time, put the weight back on? Do you still want to lose weight but no longer believe that any diet will really work for you?

We know exactly how you feel. We also know that we have empowered many to lose weight and keep it off—for good.

At the Rice Diet Program, we, a registered dietitian and a cardiologist, have helped thousands of Ricers (our affectionate name for the participants who come to our program) lose weight. Some come to lose 100 or 200 pounds. Others come to us for help losing 20 pounds they've put on since stopping a sport, having a baby, or entering middle age. The reasons people gain weight vary enormously, but the way they can lose weight and maintain their goal is actually quite simple: the Rice Diet Program.

The Rice Diet Program was established in Durham, North Carolina, over sixty years ago, and since that time the Rice Diet's results are well documented by extensive studies on hundreds of people, and impressive data on thousands. It is the most medically sound program for weight reduction, and the fastest. So whether you want to lose 10 pounds or 200, the Rice Diet will show you how to lose weight safely and quickly. The Diet will also cleanse and detox your body, ridding it of excess sodium, water weight, and other toxins from both processed foods and the environment.

Here's how it works:

• As a low-sodium diet, the Rice Diet dramatically limits salt and all other sodium-rich ingredients. Salt, like refined sugar, is an appetite stimulant. Since you will be eating mostly fresh, whole foods and dramatically reducing processed foods, you will sharply reduce your major sources of sodium (salt). Without this extra sodium, you lose not only water weight but weight associated with overeating. Ricers often say that salt works like sugar to trigger overeating; with so little salt, they rid themselves of yet another trigger that stimulates eating!

• As a low-fat diet, the Rice Diet limits saturated fats and instead relies upon carbohydrates as the main source of food. You will be eating a lot of fruits, vegetables, grains, and beans—all whole foods that contain a lot of fiber. This high fiber cleanses your body and fills you up so you feel full more quickly with less food and calories.

• People feel satiated, rarely hungry, and lose weight faster than any other whole-food diet because they easily limit calories. It's a challenge to eat 1,500 calories on this diet.

The result? You lose weight—fast and safely.

Though the rapidity of your weight loss depends on your age, sex, initial weight, and ability to exercise, men lose an average of 30 pounds and women an average of 19 pounds in the first four weeks. Over a period of months, a weight loss of 2½ to 3½ pounds per week (or ⅓ to ½ pound per day) is very doable. You will lose even more by gradually increasing your amount of exercise. It is very common for Ricers to lose several pounds per week. One Ricer lost over a pound a day, for a total of 217 pounds in less than seven months. As S.S. said, "In 1980, while in residence in Durham for ten months, I lost

150 pounds under the supervision of the Rice Diet staff. Here it is fifteen years later. I have maintained my weight at 115 pounds all these years. It is the hardest thing that I have ever done. My life began again when I lost the weight. This is not to say that you don't have problems when you're fat; it's an illness that shows on the outside. It's all consuming and distracts you from the real problem—the unresolved issues within you. I can't hold my fat accountable anymore, but I wouldn't have it any other way."

Another young man told us, "My great-grandfather came to the Rice Diet Program in the 1940s to lose weight after a heart attack, so I always knew about the place. I had gotten to the point where I was embarrassed to go out with friends because I was always the largest one there and felt uncomfortable. I knew that if I did not do something about it then, that it would only get worse and I would not end up living the long, healthy life that everyone desires. When I arrived at the 'Rice House' [the popular nickname for the Program's home base] on May 9, 2000, I was twenty-one years old, had a size 56 waist, wore a size 6X shirt, and weighed 359 pounds. Now, August 1, 2001, I am twenty-two years old, I have a size 36 waist, wear a size Large or XL shirt, and weigh an incredible 215 pounds. I cannot say enough good things about the Rice Diet. People and places come into your life for a reason; this place came into my life for reasons that I will continue to discover throughout the long life it has given me back."

One of the unique and ingenious truths of the Rice Diet is that you can tailor it to your needs. We have designed three phases of the diet: Phase One focuses on cleansing your body to ready it for true, lasting weight loss; Phase Two guides you to lose the weight; and Phase Three shows you how to maintain your weight loss. We give you the guidelines and the portion sizes; and then you decide on how you want to do the three phases in order to reach your weight loss goals. You are also free to eat any food you want—presuming that it does not cause you health problems. You are able to select from all the food groups: grains, legumes (beans), fruits, vegetables, fish and meats, dairy, and fats (preferably olive oil).

There are three other keys to making the Rice Diet work for you:

becoming a mindful eater by learning about nutrition, relaxing and making time for yourself through exercise and other mindful activities, and by creating support in your community. When Ricers put these pieces of the weight loss puzzle into place, they are pretty much guaranteed to lose the weight they desire and maintain their weight loss. Our results are the best we've seen for long-term success: 43 percent of our participants maintained their weight loss, or lost even more, after six years back home!

Within days of starting the Rice Diet, you will feel remarkably better: more clearheaded, more energetic, more at peace with yourself. You will know that the Diet is working for you not just because you are losing weight, but because you suddenly feel unburdened from living—and eating—in a way that hasn't worked for you. This is when something magical happens: When you are freed from the grip of processed food's excess fat, sodium, and sugar, your weight loss inspires you to explore your "inner healing" tools that heal at the root level, and you discover that you truly have the power to actualize your goal weight, as well as other lifelong dreams.

We have watched these transformations again and again with Ricers at the program. When people finally learn to control their eating and achieve lasting weight loss, they do so with the understanding that they can choose to think differently—and more positively—about their bodies. And as a result they begin to expect more from their futures than they ever realized was possible. This is a diet that has the simplicity and the scientific support to give you the tools to cleanse your body of toxins, lose weight in the short- and long-term, and give you the power to actualize all your lifelong dreams. It is this combination that can lead you to change your life. Now what's stopping you from becoming a Ricer?

# CHAPTER ONE

# HOW TODAY'S RICE DIET PROGRAM CAME TO BE

*Whenever a new discovery is reported to the scientific world they say first, "It is probably not true." Thereafter, when the truth of the new proposition has been demonstrated beyond question, they say, "Yes, it may be true but it is not important." Finally, when sufficient time has elapsed to fully evidence its importance, they say, "Yes, surely it is important, but it is no longer new."*

—MONTAIGNE

It's true that the Rice Diet can help you lose weight, improve your health, and better the quality of your life, but it's how the Diet offers this transformation that has people coming to our clinic from all over the world. Simply put, the Rice Diet is not just an eating plan. It's a physical, emotional, and spiritual program that will change the way you live, giving you new vitality, energy, and longevity. People who come to the Rice Diet Program experience the three-dimensionality of the diet, but Kitty—my wife and co-director—and I feel compelled to share this experience—and opportunity—with all of you who have not had the chance to visit us here in Durham, North Carolina.

In 1939, a German-born, Duke University physician, Dr. Walter Kempner, advised a thirty-three-year-old female patient with hypertension, renal disease, and associated symptoms to follow a diet of only rice and fruit for two weeks upon being discharged from the hospital. Speaking in a German accent, Dr. Kempner was especially difficult for this native North Carolinian patient to understand. And while she understood that she could eat rice, and she did that faithfully, she did not understand his instructions to return in two weeks.

Finally, two months later she returned to Dr. Kempner for a follow-up examination, and her results were amazing. Her blood pressure was reduced from 190/120 to 124/84. This was incredibly significant because at this time high blood pressure medications had not yet been invented. In addition, the bleeding in her eye had healed, and there was a substantial decrease in her heart size. When Dr. Kempner realized that the diet could produce these dramatic results and could be used over longer periods of time, the Rice Diet Program was born and became his mission.

Excited by his patient's success, Dr. Kempner began prescribing prolonged diet therapy to other patients with renal disease and hypertension with equally positive results. In 1944, he presented his clinical findings to the American Heart Association meeting in Chicago. The results were revolutionary. Dr. Kempner documented improvements in kidney dysfunction, hypertension, cholesterol levels, and cardiovascular disease. Three years later, he reported the disappearance of signs and symptoms of congestive heart failure. By 1958, Dr. Kempner had proved that dietary therapy could reduce or eliminate the need for insulin therapy for people suffering from Type 2 diabetes.

Dr. Kempner's patients noted one other remarkable effect: It was almost impossible for them *not* to lose weight following the diet. Dr. Kempner had discovered another population he could treat with his Rice Diet: women and men who were overweight or obese. The Rice Diet, which was affiliated with Duke University at that time, began emerging as the benchmark for all other diet programs. Soon it became known nationally and internationally as a weight loss plan, and the program's popularity soared. Since that time, the Rice Diet has become known for treatment of obesity, and its hometown of Durham, North Carolina, has developed a reputation as the "diet capital of the world."

When I first started working with Dr. Kempner and his colleague Dr. Barbara Newborg in 1983, there was no "Program" in the traditional sense of lectures, groups, or supervised exercise. There was simply an eating plan and a medical check-in. Participants came to the Rice House for breakfast and met with staff to have their weights, blood pressure, and, if necessary, blood sugars checked. The doctors made recommendations about medications, exercise, and diet. After breakfast the Rice House closed. If the patient wanted to see the medical staff after 10 A.M., they went to the clinic. The Rice House reopened for two hours for lunch and dinner, but otherwise patients were on their own. Dr. Kempner suggested that they take a walk in the morning and a nap in the afternoon. That was the extent of the "Program." It was simply the phenomenal results as well as Dr. Kempner's larger-than-life personality and his steadfast belief in what he was doing that kept patients committed to the diet.

At this time in the history of the Rice Diet, I was a staff physician. Part of my job was to talk to prospective patients on the phone and describe the program. Dutifully, I would tell them to show up at the Rice House for their meals, see their doctor to have their daily workup, and simply take it easy. The people at the other end of the phone would take in this information and then ask me what everyone did the rest of the day. They wanted to know what to do with all that free time. I wasn't sure, but I assured them that by the end of the first week, patients reported that they didn't have a free minute.

The more I pondered this common question, the more I began to realize that patients did one of two things with all that free time: they got bored and either started figuring out why they were doing the Rice Diet in the first place, or they found ways to distract themselves. I could see that this "boredom" time seemed to be having a positive impact on the participants' emotional and psychological lives: they were losing weight like gangbusters; they seemed happy; and they were feeling better than they had in years. But at some point, the boredom caught up with them: they began to slow down—they either stopped losing weight, or gained back one or two pounds, and they were forced to look inward. They asked themselves questions, such as "Why am I here? What am I doing? Who am I?" It was clear to me that it was the so-called boredom time that enabled these questions to surface and brought participants to a critical turning point. Some of them would say in frustration, "I just want to be thin!" Years later I would say, "Of course you do, but that thin person is inside of you. Just look inside."

As I began to see people doing this self-exploration on their own, I realized that they might benefit further from psychological or therapeutic help. Though trained as an internist, Dr. Kempner was quite a good psychiatrist and was already helping patients deal with emotional issues. He could go straight to the cause of a patient's stress and counsel him or her on how he or she might reduce or eliminate it. He also told patients that they needed to be "completely selfish," which was pretty startling advice, but I realized that he was talking about priorities and taking care of yourself. Confucius said something like, "First take care of yourself. If you could do that you might be able to take care of another and if you could do that you might be able to take care of a family and if everybody could do that the world would be better."

It began to dawn on me that most of our patients had been so busy taking care of someone or something else that they had no time to take care of themselves. Doing the Rice Diet was often the first time many of them had made the choice to take care of themselves.

It was around this time that Kitty came into my life. Her joyful, tenacious intelligence, and her belief in people's ability to change their lives for the better was present as much in her personality as it was in her work as a dietitian. Seeing both her success working with patients in cardiac rehab as well as in changing their lives through nutrition, I convinced Dr. Kempner to hire her. I believed strongly that she would be an enormous asset to the Rice Diet, and I was right.

Immediately, Kitty began nutritional talks, helping all participants doing the Rice Diet understand why they were eating the foods they were eating. At the same time, she not only empowered the participants to find health through weight loss and motivated them to seek self-exploration and inner healing, she also inspired me to open my eyes to how necessary such inner examination is for everyone, including me. Kitty suggested we model this part of the diet process on a 12-Step program, offering participants groups that followed the book, *The 12 Steps.*

You might think that I should have learned about 12-Step programs in medical school, but it wasn't part of the curriculum. At any rate, I realized that most patients who came to us had implicitly done the first three steps: (1) they realized that they had a problem that they could not manage; (2) they believed that there was a way to get help; and (3) they turned the management of the problem to a higher power.

Using Dr. Kempner's approach as our inspiration, Kitty and I began to put into place a program that led people to take further steps, enabling them to do some inner examination of their lives, including their eating behavior, and slowly but surely integrate skills for living the diet outside of our clinic in Durham. Indeed, it turns out that many participants were already doing step four (i.e., making a searching and fearless moral inventory of themselves) when they got bored and started their self-examinations. Patients were responding well to the opportunity our 12-Step-like groups gave them to explore in a safe and honest environment their struggle with food and the resulting feelings of shame that challenged their weight loss success. With Kitty at the helm, we looked in the direction of personal recovery in order to help people lose weight and keep it off for good.

When Dr. Kempner retired and Kitty and I assumed day-to-day operations of the Rice Diet Clinic, we continued expanding the program, offering more opportunities for those ready to explore a deeper connection to their bodies, minds, and spirits. We soon added yoga, and an increasing number of scheduled activities, including meditation and mindfulness exercises. We strengthened the community at the Rice House, giving participants many opportunities to gather, share experiences, ask questions, and mull over their own thoughts and feelings with like-minded, encouraging listeners. When we saw how much the community helped people maintain the diet, I finally understood what Dr. Kempner had told me long before: "The patients are each other's therapists." In short, that is the story of how today's Rice Diet Program came to be.

Our mutual desire is to inspire the readers of this book to maximize their life's potential. Through decades of teaching, writing, and sharing in heart-to-heart groups, we are not only wed to one another but also to the mission of inspiring our participants to live their lives to the fullest. Although most Rice Diet Program participants come to lose weight fast and safely, our main interest is that they take this opportunity to truly know who they are and, thus, achieve long-term weight loss success and healthy, happy lives.

# INSPIRATIONAL CORNER

John is a big guy, nice-looking, carrying 290-plus pounds on his 6'4" frame—about the same as when he was playing high school football. He has brown hair and a mustache and the direct, thoughtful gaze of someone who thinks about what he says before he says it. There's nothing particularly remarkable about him—until you hear what he's been doing for the last fourteen months: Since enrolling in the Rice Diet Program on January 11, 2000, John has lost over 360 pounds.

He is amazingly matter-of-fact about his feat. "A lot of people ask me for secrets. Well, there is no secret," he says. "It's just a matter of doing it. I've worked hard all my life. This is just another hard job to get done. For me there's not any other choice. If you're not going to do it, you might as well go home."

John was born in 1950 in a small farming community of four or five hundred. It's a stone's throw from where he and his brothers now run the family farms. Hog farming is hardly an armchair job; surely it was hard to meet the physical demands, carrying so much weight? John considers this for a moment, then shakes his head. "My weight was always up and down. Most of the time I never let it bother me. I played a lot of basketball a few years ago, softball for about fifteen years, really very successfully. I was about 350 pounds and accustomed to carrying weight around. But the last two or three years it got progressively worse. I was able to haul grain, but the actual physical work, feeding the hogs and things like that, became very, very difficult. Jobs that shouldn't have been that tough turned into major challenges."

Then about a year and a half before he came to us, John

injured his knee, which further restricted his mobility, and the weight began piling on. He tried different kinds of diets, with mixed success. John's increasing immobility began to affect his social and work life. He quit going to the town tavern where the farmers gather to talk and keep in touch. Sitting at the tables made his knee hurt, and even walking across the parking lot from the truck had become a challenge. Then there was the end-of-harvest turkey barbecue, he recalls, when he found himself unable to get up from the picnic table without help from bystanders. A wince of pain crosses his face at the memory. "You get to the point where you just don't want to fight it anymore," he says. "You decide it's a hopeless case."

So what changed his mind, and how did he end up at the Rice House? "I think what set things in motion was when I fell off my bed. All of a sudden I woke up and was falling to the floor, and I thought I'd broken my foot. I lay there and thought, if I have to get a cast on, I won't even be able to care for myself." He was so scared of the possibility that he put off going to the doctor for several days, just sitting around the house hurting and feeling sorry for himself. Finally, his brothers came to the house and confronted him.

So John, with his brother and sister-in-law and their two sons, made the two-day drive in two cars, so that he could keep one in Durham. "It was a terribly long drive," he remembers. "I wasn't very comfortable, sitting there all day like that. We got here and checked into the motel, and the next morning we went to the Rice Diet Clinic." At the clinic, the medical staff weighed John, gave him a physical, ran some tests—and were amazed. "I remember the doctors looking at my blood tests and just kind of shaking their heads," John says, with a small smile. "The amazing thing is that my blood pressure was really just about normal and my cholesterol was 152 and my blood sugar was okay. It was just astonishing that I was in the health I was in, not diabetic. But it would have been just a matter of time, I'm sure. Basically, I'm a perfectly healthy guy, I just weighed too much."

However, that initial clinical assessment held a nasty surprise for John. After not having weighed himself for years, he watched in horror as the scales mounted to 651 pounds. "I just couldn't believe it! I remember I lay in my room the first two or three nights and I cried. I kept saying 'It's impossible!' I had thought I could come out here, lose maybe 100 pounds, and be in pretty good shape. But 300 pounds! It didn't seem like anything that could possibly be done. But I was here, so I thought I would give it a try."

Initially, the doctors restricted John's exercise to lying on the floor with his feet up, in order to reduce the edema in his legs. On the diet, he began losing weight immediately, a pound or two every day. After a couple of weeks, he began walking in the swimming pool, increasing his distance every day. He then joined a water aerobics class. After a while, a fellow participant persuaded him to try the exercise bike.

"The first week was living hell. Getting used to the seat of the bike was just terrible! But I started doing that, and still doing the water aerobics. And every day I felt better." On the bike, John increased his distance to 20 miles a day. About three months after enrolling, he had dropped 150 pounds, so he added weight lifting to his regimen, alternating it with the bike. Then a few months later he began trail walking.

Somehow, listening to John talk about his amazing self-transformation in that calm, considering voice, you could almost believe it was easy—but he doesn't encourage any illusions about that. It was a long, hard row to hoe. And he's quick to acknowledge the factors that made success possible for him, the sources of strength both internal and external. Especially, he says, his spirits and his determination were buoyed up by the attitude of the Rice House staff and by the other participants.

"One thing I want to make sure people know is that if they come here and follow the program, stick to it, it'll work. It's as good as you want to make it. The people here are so helpful, so great.

"I think the secret is to try to have a lot of interests in life. In this program you find people who are positive and those who sit around and feel sorry for themselves and don't like the food. It's your choice if you want to be here or not. But as long as you're here, spending the money and the time, you might as well try to be positive. My brother, who's into tai chi, always says, you don't want to hang around people who take away from your chi, your power, or your energy. I try to stay away from people like that."

After more than a year's hard work every day, John achieved more than he ever thought possible. He started to make plans to go home for the first time in fifteen months, to leave the Rice House, which he calls a second home and a second family. "It's going to be hard to leave here in a lot of ways, because I've made a lot of friends here. I'm safe here. I know what I can do. As long as I stick with the program there's nothing to worry about. And another thing, everybody telling you how good you look! I guess compared to the way you were, you do look good. But you've got to take it with a grain of salt, because you don't want to get too happy with yourself. You've still got a lot of work to do."

All modesty. All caution. John is a true champ, but it's hard to get him to pat himself on the back. Finally, after a little needling, he flashes a rare, broad grin—sort of like that springtime prairie sun warming up. "Yeah, I am really proud of myself." Then he adds, "But I'll tell you more in a year. I've got to see that I can keep it off. . . ."

Since John returned home and resumed farming five years ago, he continues to follow the Rice Diet and has lost an additional 55 pounds. He tells us that he does not feel that he is on a diet, but "this is just the way I eat."

# CHAPTER TWO

# THE RICE DIET

*The doctor of the future will give no medicines, but will interest his patients in the care of the human frame, in diet and the prevention of disease.*

—Thomas Edison

# A NEW *DIETA*

As we mentioned above, the Rice Diet is not just an eating plan. Rather, it is what we call a *dieta*, which comes from the Greek word *diaita*, meaning way of life. We believe that in order to lose weight and keep it off, you must truly change the way you live. Now, before you get scared that we are asking you to turn your lives upside down, take a breath (actually, we will be encouraging you to take a lot of breaths throughout the course of this book), and answer these questions for yourself:

• **Do you want to lose weight?**

• **Do you *hope* that it is possible?**

• **Are you ready to create a new *dieta?***

If you answered yes to these three questions, know that the Rice Diet offers you:

• **a clear simple diet to follow**

• **a way to change the way you think about food**

• **techniques to guide you to rediscover yourself and your dreams**

• **support and encouragement as you begin this life-changing process**

There are four essential steps that guarantee success. The first step is doing the diet itself. The Rice Diet consists of three phases, is astonishingly simple, and can be done almost anywhere. With the carefully calibrated intake of calories and low-sodium foods, your appetite is easily satisfied. Phase One, which lasts one week, begins with one day of the Basic Rice Diet, consisting of grains and fruits. For the other six days of the week, you add in vegetables, regular (i.e. *not* low-sodium) whole-grain cereal or bread, and some nonfat dairy, preferably soymilk. The focus or goal of Phase One is to detox your body and mind and prepare it for lasting weight loss in Phase Two. As you will see in Chapter 6, there is a lot of freedom to make your own choices and adapt the diet to your liking once you are familiar with your routine and are comfortable with the amount of weight you are losing.

In Phase Two, your focus becomes lasting weight loss. You will begin each week with one day of the Basic Rice Diet, and then do five days of fruit, grains, and veggies, some nonfat dairy (soy, grain, or cow milk), regular whole-grain cereal or bread, and on the seventh day (or day of your choice), you will add in one protein source, such as fish, more non-fat dairy, or organic eggs. If you are allergic to these high protein sources, or really prefer other lean-meat choices, check your cholesterol before and several weeks after making these additions. In Phase Two you will eat slightly more sodium because vegetables, fish, and other animal products contain more naturally occurring sodium than grains or fruits, and it allows more calories because of the 200-calorie addition of the protein group.

Once you have reached your goals, you move into Phase Three, our maintenance plan, which is the same as Phase Two, but adds more choices and more opportunities to eat protein, and to enjoy a little flexibility with the sodium. That's the diet!

The second step is becoming a mindful eater. We have watched hundreds of women and men change their *dieta*, or way of life, not simply by following our instructions and eating the food prescribed on the Rice Diet, but by integrating the nutritional information about the foods they are eating. When people understand what they are eating—carbs, protein, fats, fiber, sodium, and so on—they take the first step to becoming conscious and aware of food and what it means to eat well. Becoming a mindful eater starts with a basic understanding of the nutritional content of food and leads to a heightened awareness of the process of eating. In other words, if you understand what you are eating, you are more likely to make food choices that actually promote weight loss and health. It's that simple. But hold on, there's more to help deepen your commitment to the diet.

The third step asks participants to make time for themselves each day to rest. In rest, you give yourself the opportunity to think, to feel, and come to know and listen to yourself more clearly. Most participants who come to us have not spent one minute meditating on themselves and their lives. The thinking and feeling we are inviting them to explore is not the common practice of fretting and worrying about our family or business, but learning to breathe deeply and observe what comes up; to be with and observe our thoughts and feelings. This step of the Rice Diet Program shows you how to become aware and observant of, rather than obsessive and attached to, your worries, stresses, and concerns about life, so that you can truly relax and have time for yourself.

This "self time" is what enables you to ask yourself questions such as, "Why do I want to lose weight? What do I want from my life? Where am I going? Who am I, really?" Through mindful activities such as meditation, yoga, tai chi, journalizing, and exercising, you will gain insight and clarity of mind.

Regular exercise is also a powerful way to create such quiet time; it also maximizes the benefits of the Rice Diet. To succeed at losing weight and keeping it off, everyone needs regular quiet time to connect with their inner selves. These mindfulness tools will help you succeed with the diet because they put you in touch with your own power and potential to create the life you want. With these two steps—becoming a mindful eater and making time to rest—people begin to change their *dieta* at a deep, emotional level and assure their commitment to the diet, their weight loss, and the transformation of their lives.

The fourth step offers ways to create the support you need to stick to the diet and your new lifestyle. One of the biggest challenges with maintaining a healthy diet over time is that most everyone you know is eating less-than-health-promoting foods. It's challenging to be different. With this in mind, we guide participants to find support in their communities, establish nurturing relationships, and form new groups of companions or friends for exercise and introspection. You can find others who are committed to taking better care of themselves at health clubs, at churches and synagogues, in cardiac rehabilitation programs, with special interest groups such as vegetarians, in yoga and meditation classes, on the Internet, in Anonymous groups, and in group therapy. See Appendix B for other professional support services and outreach facilities.

While healthier foods are more available than a decade ago, it requires a conscious choice to buy and enjoy them. Fortunately, eating less and more healthfully, while it takes a commitment, doesn't take any more time. To maintain a healthier lifestyle, we need not just a commitment to the diet, but a commitment to taking time for ourselves on a regular basis.

# THE THREE PHASES

Unless you try it, you probably cannot imagine how astonishingly simple, straightforward, and easy the Rice Diet is. The foods are delicious and can be found everywhere. The directions are so simple you have virtually nothing to memorize. The portion sizes are standardized, so that once you are introduced to them, you will be able to eyeball almost all amounts without having to continue to weigh or measure. You will be able to do the Rice Diet almost anywhere you live or anywhere you travel.

We have developed three phases of the diet so that your body has a chance to cleanse itself of excess sodium, toxins, and water weight (Phase One), lose unwanted pounds according to your personal goals (Phase Two), and maintain your new weight (Phase Three). As you move through all three phases you will naturally become more mindful of what, why, and how you are eating; this shift is pivotal for you to become more conscious of what your body wants and needs to lose weight and stay healthy.

Although the three phases gradually increase from just under 1,000 to over 1,200 calories per day, you don't have to worry about keeping track of your calories. Rather, we have defined serving sizes for each food group so that all you need to do is select foods from the menus listed under each of the phases and in Chapter Nine and follow the serving size guidelines indicated. As you move from Phase One to Phases Two and Three, the foods naturally become more complicated, as food groups are mixed for taste, variation, and to keep your creative needs met for the long haul. But again, you will not have to worry about counting calories. Instead, you will have clear guidelines that incorporate the amount of calories appropriate for you whether you are in detox mode (Phase One), weight loss mode (Phase Two), or maintenance mode (Phase Three).

The diet is essentially a low-sodium, low-fat diet. You do not add any salt to your food and we suggest eating no processed foods that contain a lot of sodium, although some very low-sodium processed foods are shared in the Healthy Grocery List found on page 42. We recommend that Ricers at home average between 500 and 1,000 milligrams of sodium each day, with a minimum of 300 milligrams per day. Basically, the Phase One and Two guidelines in this book will provide you with 300 to 500 milligrams per day; in Phase Three you will average between 500 and 1,000 milligrams. A general rule of thumb is to not add salt to your food or use on a regular basis processed foods or products to which sodium has been added, unless you are choosing to enjoy them in insuring your daily 300 milligram sodium minimum.

We also recommend that every day you choose a regular (not low-sodium) whole-grain cereal, such as Kashi or Health Valley, or

# BEFORE BEGINNING
# THE RICE DIET

It is important to check with your physician prior to
beginning any diet, especially if you are taking any
medications. Due to the rapid weight loss with the Rice Diet,
it is important to consult with your physician before reducing
your fat, sodium, and calories. You may be on medication
that will need to be altered or discontinued before changing
your diet, and your doctor is the best person to help you do
this. Do not make any changes in your medication regimen
without your physician's advice. Since many physicians and
health care professionals are unfamiliar with the impact of a
truly low-sodium diet, you should point out the low-sodium
content of the Rice Diet to your doctor. Feel free, as well,
to refer your physician to the Rice Diet Program and we
will be happy to be of assistance. We can be reached at
www.ricediet.com.

regular (not low-sodium) bread such as Ezekiel 4:9, along with one
serving of dairy. The cereal or bread plus dairy, along with the 100
milligrams of sodium found naturally in grains, fruits, and vegetables, will satisfy the 300 milligrams of sodium you need each day.
Throughout the discussion of the Rice Diet, we have focused on
such low-sodium options. We do this so that you can become familiar with them for enjoyment throughout, but particularly for the Basic Rice Diet day (one day a week) and for when you start adding
higher sodium options in Phases Two and Three. For instance, later
you might want to use the low-sodium version of Ezekiel 4:9 if you
are making a bruschetta with olive oil and a freshly grated Parmesan
and red-pepper-flake topping. Thus, you learn to use primarily low-

sodium items, with very few higher-sodium items, so that you can keep your sodium intake between 500 and 1,000 milligram per day.

Finally, if dairy and cereal are not your thing and bread inspires cravings, you can get to your 300-milligram-sodium minimum by flavoring your grains or vegetables with a few olives, anchovies, or capers, all of which contain sodium. But remember to read your food labels and keep your consumption of these higher-sodium options to less than 200 milligrams per day.

And given that the diet is made up mostly of whole grains, fruits, vegetables, beans, dairy, and fish (and increasing amounts of dairy, seafood, olive oil, skinned poultry, and lean meat, if desired), you will naturally be eating a low-fat diet. So don't worry: If you stick to the diet plan, it is not necessary to count calories or calculate percentage of calories coming from fat.

# A QUICK-AND-EASY VIEW OF THE RICE DIET

## PORTIONS

| | |
|---|---|
| 1 starch = | ⅓ cup cooked rice or dried beans or ½ cup cooked grains, pasta, or starchy vegetables (potatoes, corn, green peas, yams) or 1 slice bread or ¼ to 1 cup cereal |
| 1 non-fat dairy = | 1 cup non-fat soy or grain milk (calcium fortified), or cow's milk or yogurt |
| 1 vegetable = | ½ cup cooked or 1 cup raw vegetable |
| 1 fruit = | 1 medium size fruit or 1 cup of grapes or 1 cup of cut fruit |

Condiments: No-salt added seasoning and herbs are okay.

1 teaspoon of maple syrup or honey per day is okay.

**ANY GRAIN, ANY FRUIT, ANY VEGETABLE WITH NO SALT, NO FAT ADDED IS OKAY!**

# PHASE ONE

**FOR 1 DAY A WEEK: Basic Rice Diet**

BREAKFAST: 2 starches & 2 fruits

LUNCH: 2 starches & 2 fruits

DINNER: 2 starches & 2 fruits

---

**FOR 6 DAYS A WEEK: Lacto-Vegetarian Rice Diet**

BREAKFAST: 1 starch, 1 non-fat dairy, & 1 fruit

LUNCH: 3 starches, 3 vegetables & 1 fruit

DINNER: 3 starches, 3 vegetables & 1 fruit

### SAMPLES

| ONE STARCH | ONE VEGETABLE | ONE FRUIT | ONE DAIRY |
|---|---|---|---|
| ½ cup cooked grain or starchy vegetable | ½ cup tomato sauce | 1 medium apple | 1 cup soy or grain milk |
| ¼ to 1 cup cereal | ½ cup steamed broccoli | 3 prunes | 1 cup nonfat yogurt |
| ⅓ cup cooked rice or dried beans, or peas | 1 cup spinach (raw) salad | ½ banana | ½ cup dry curd cottage cheese |
| 1 slice bread | 1 cup raw carrots | 2 tablespoons raisins | 1 cup skim milk |

(Remember, these samples are one serving portion and you often get two or three servings in a meal, as shown above.)

# PHASE TWO

**FOR 1 DAY A WEEK: Basic Rice Diet**

BREAKFAST: 2 starches & 2 fruits

LUNCH: 2 starches & 2 fruits

DINNER: 2 starches & 2 fruits

---

**FOR 5 DAYS A WEEK: Lacto-Vegetarian Rice Diet**

BREAKFAST: 1 starch, 1 non-fat dairy & 1 fruit

LUNCH: 3 starches, 3 vegetables & 1 fruit

DINNER: 3 starches, 3 vegetables & 1 fruit

---

**FOR 1 DAY A WEEK: Vegetarian Plus Rice Diet**

BREAKFAST: 2 starches & 1 fruit

LUNCH: 3 starches, 3 vegetables & 1 fruit

DINNER: 3 starches, 3 protein (or 2 dairy), 3 vegetables & 1 fruit

## SAMPLES

| ONE STARCH | ONE VEGETABLE | ONE FRUIT | ONE DAIRY | ONE FISH PROTEIN |
|---|---|---|---|---|
| ⅓ cup cooked rice or beans | ½ cup tomato sauce | 1 cup melon | 1 cup skim milk | 1 ounce cooked flounder |
| ¾ cup Health Valley cereal | ½ cup steamed broccoli | 1 cup strawberries | 1 cup soy or grain milk | 1 ounce cooked salmon |
| ½ cup cooked steel-cut oats | 1 cup spinach (raw) salad | ½ banana | ½ cup dry curd cottage cheese (<65 mg sodium) | 1 ounce canned kippers or sardines |
| ½ cup starchy vegetable | 1 cup raw carrots | 2 tablespoons raisins | 1 cup nonfat yogurt | 1 ounce canned tuna (¼ cup) |

# PHASE THREE

### FOR 1 DAY A WEEK: Basic Rice Diet

BREAKFAST: 2 starches & 2 fruits

LUNCH: 2 starches & 2 fruits

DINNER: 2 starches & 2 fruits

---

### FOR 4 DAYS A WEEK: Lacto-Vegetarian Rice Diet

BREAKFAST: 1 starch, 1 nonfat dairy & 1 fruit

LUNCH: 3 starches, 3 vegetables & 1 fruit

DINNER: 3 starches, 3 vegetables & 1 fruit

---

### FOR 2 DAYS A WEEK: Vegetarian Plus Rice Diet

BREAKFAST: 2 starches & 1 fruit

LUNCH: 3 starches, 3 vegetables & 1 fruit

DINNER: 3 starches, 3 proteins (or 2 dairy), 3 vegetables & 1 fruit

### SAMPLES

| ONE STARCH | ONE VEGETABLE | ONE FRUIT | ONE DAIRY | ONE PROTEIN |
|---|---|---|---|---|
| ⅓ cup cooked rice or beans | ½ cup tomato sauce | 1 cup blueberries | 1 cup skim milk | ¼ cup cooked beans |
| ½ cup starchy vegetable | ½ cup steamed broccoli | ¼ cup dried apricots | 1 cup soy or grain milk | 1 ounce cooked salmon |
| 1 slice bread | 1 cup spinach (raw) salad | ½ banana | ½ cup dry curd cottage cheese (<65 mg sodium) | 1 ounce chicken breast skinned |
| ⅓ cup Nature's Path Granola | 1 cup raw carrots | 2 tablespoons raisins | ¼ cup grated parmesan cheese | 1 cooked egg or 3 egg whites |

# PHASE ONE: DETOX

In Phase One you will be eating one day of the Basic Rice Diet (a limited amount of grains and fruit) and six days of the Lacto-Vegetarian Rice Diet (grains, beans, vegetables, fruits, and some dairy). The overall goal of Phase One is to cleanse and detox your body's system of excess water weight (most people carry more than 5 to 10 pounds of excess water weight), excess sodium, allergic-like symptoms from a range of potential offenders from our food supply (e.g., pesticides, fertilizers, antibiotic and growth hormone dosed animal products, and others). You will eat simple, fresh whole foods, which will also cleanse your palate and enhance your appreciation of food's natural flavor. You will receive plenty of benefits in consuming grains and fruit one day per week, and adding vegetables, beans, and organic milk (soy, grain, or cow) the other six days.

## SAMPLE MENU—PHASE ONE

### Day One: The Basic Rice Diet

| | |
|---|---|
| Breakfast: | 2 starches = 1 cup cooked oatmeal, oat bran, or steel-cut oats |
| | 2 fruits = 1 peach + 2 tablespoons raisins |
| Lunch: | 2 starches = ⅔ cup cooked rice, brown preferred |
| | 2 fruits = 1 cup pineapple chunks + 1 cup grapes |
| Dinner: | 2 starches = ⅔ cup cooked rice, brown preferred |
| | 2 fruits = 1 cup mixed berries + 1 cup melon |

## Days 2 to 7: The Lacto-Vegetarian Rice Diet

**To be enjoyed six days per week for one week.**

Breakfast:     1 starch = ½ cup grain cereal OR 1 slice toast

1 non-fat dairy = 1 cup non-fat soy, grain, or cow's milk

1 fruit = 1 peach

---

Lunch:     3 starches = 1 cup cooked rice and/or beans OR 1½ cups of any other cooked grain, pasta, or starchy vegetable

3 vegetables = 3 cups raw vegetable salad OR 1½ cups cooked broccoli

1 fruit = 1 cup fresh fruit salad

---

Dinner:     3 starches = 1 cup cooked rice and/or beans OR 1½ cups of any other cooked grain or pasta

3 vegetables = 3 cups raw OR 1½ cups cooked cabbage

1 fruit = 1 cup berries

The total calories you will consume is 6,800 per week. We recommend beginning with Phase One and doing it for one week. Sticking to Phase One for one week is best to detox and cleanse your body, refresh your palate, and retrain your neurological pathways with your more conscious food choices. You may notice that your calcium-fortified soy or grain milk or cow milk is higher in sodium than any of the whole vegetarian foods. This Phase One plan will average approximately 300 milligrams of sodium per day. If you don't consume dairy, then you need to eat 2 slices of regular bread or 200 milligrams of added sodium from another, more enjoyable source daily to ensure that you get adequate sodium.

If you do not care for any soy, grain, or cow milk straight, try blending your milk choice with some fresh or frozen fruit, cinnamon, and vanilla extract in a blender. If you still don't care for the smoothie, you can consume the desired calcium and sodium that the dairy would have offered via generous amounts of dried beans and dark green leafy vegetables, collards and kale. It is prudent and preventive to supplement with 600 to 1,000 milligrams of calcium per day, plus a general multivitamin/mineral pill, or as your physician recommends.

# PHASE TWO: LASTING WEIGHT LOSS

Now that you have cleansed and prepared your body in Phase One, you are primed and ready to continue your weight loss and appreciation for the growing number of healthy and delicious food choices to come in Phase Two. In Phase Two, you continue to do one day of the Basic Rice Diet (fruits and grains), followed by five days of grains, beans, fruit, veggies, and non-fat dairy (the Lacto-Vegetarian Rice Diet). Then on one day—of your choice, though many people choose the weekend—you add fish. If you don't care for fish, you can replace it with non-fat dairy (milk or yogurt—preferably organic soy or grain), or eggs (free-range, organic preferred), or lean meat (again, organic or free-range preferred) instead; we call this the Vegetarian Plus Rice Diet. The total calorie count increases from 6,800 per week to 7,000 per week. All foods in italics can be found in the recipe section in Chapter 9.

# SAMPLE MENUS—PHASE TWO

## Day 1: The Basic Rice Diet

**To be enjoyed no more than one day per week without our medical supervision.**

Breakfast:    2 starches = 1 cup oatmeal

2 fruits = 2 tablespoons raisins + 1 cup melon

Lunch:    2 starches = ⅔ cup cooked rice, brown preferred

2 fruits = 1 cup pineapple chunks + 1 cup melon

Dinner:    2 starches = ⅔ cup cooked rice, brown preferred

2 fruits = 1 cup mixed berries + 1 cup grapes

## Days 2 to 6: The Lacto-Vegetarian Rice Diet

**To be enjoyed five days per week until weight and health goals are met.**

Breakfast:    1 starch = ½ cup grain cereal OR 1 slice toast

1 non-fat dairy = 1 cup non-fat soy or grain or cow's milk

1 fruit = 1 cup fresh berries

1 fruit = 2 tablespoons dried cherries or 1 tablespoon all-fruit jam

Lunch:    3 starches = 1 cup cooked rice/beans OR 1½ cups of any other cooked grain or pasta

1 vegetable = ½ cup *Tomato Sauce*

2 vegetables + 1 fruit = 2½ cups *Spinach and Mandarin Orange Salad* with 2 tablespoons *Balsamic Dressing*

Dinner:    2 starches = ⅔ cup cooked rice

1 starch = ¾ cup *Split Pea Soup*

2 vegetables = 1 cup steamed broccoli

Dinner (*cont.*):     1 vegetable = 1 cup *Cucumber and Red Pepper Salad*

1 fruit = 1 cup fresh melon

## Day 7: The Vegetarian Plus Rice Diet

**This is the same as the Lacto-Vegetarian Rice Diet + Fish or more Non-fat Dairy (an approximate 200 calorie addition).**

Breakfast:     2 starches = 1 cup cooked steel-cut oats (with cinnamon)

1 fruit = ½ banana

Lunch:     2 starches = ⅔ cup Black Pearl rice

2 starches = ⅔ cup *Black Beans 'n Garlic*

2 vegetables = 1 cup *Creamed Spinach*

1 vegetable = *Baby Greens with Roasted Bell Peppers*

1 fruit = 1 cup grapes, frozen

Dinner:     3 meats = *Crispy Flounder*

1 starch = ½ cup *Southwestern Corn*

1 starch = ½ cup *Garlic Red Skin Potatoes*

1 vegetable = 1 cup tossed salad with *Balsamic Dressing*

2 vegetables = 1 cup *Bok Choy*

1 fruit = 1 orange or 2 clementines

The length of Phase Two depends on how much weight you want to lose. Following this eating plan and coupling it with a regular exercise routine (see Chapter 5 for specifics), you will, on average, lose about 3.5 pounds per week, or 14 pounds per month.

Many conscious eaters think of both foods and calories on a weekly basis—giving themselves the freedom to add calories and specific foods on the days when they really want them. Often people begin the week (on Mondays) with fruits and grains and end the week with their choice of fish, nonfat dairy or eggs (and later lean meat or poultry, if desired)—this works to celebrate your weekend after eating more sparingly throughout the week—but it's not helpful to think of foods as "bad" or "good."

Once you have reached either your weight loss goal or health goal, you are ready to move into Phase Three, the Maintenance Diet. Most people do not experience hunger while on the program, but at home you may find your routines or stressful environmental stimuli inspire a desire to snack. You may miss your traditional 4 P.M. snack, and find that saving a fruit from lunch is much more enjoyable mid-afternoon than earlier. Or, if you really prefer those fresh tomatoes that are coming out of the garden, enjoy. At 25 calories per cup, extra vegetables are definitely the best caloric choice out there. This is your *dieta;* whatever works for you is what will be best—just keep your journal (see Chapter 6) and read the clues.

# PHASE THREE: MAINTENANCE

Reaching Phase Three is a major accomplishment. You have lost your desired amount of weight, you feel lighter, leaner, and more centered within yourself. Phase Three is all about helping you live the *dieta:* maintain your optimal weight and continue to feel healthier, stronger, and more energetic. In terms of food choices, Phase Three is the same as Phase Two but continues to add more calories (200 more per week until you stop losing weight), and you can also add some other types of food, including tofu (firm), cheese (as a condiment on top of pasta, for example), eggs, nuts and/or seeds, olives, olive oil (when you get into these higher fat and sodium-rich foods watch your volume), and seafood, lean meat, or poultry, among other protein sources. Again, in Phase Three you will encounter more food choices and more diversity as food groups are mixed in creative, delicious recipes. And don't worry about calories—the recipes account for accurate portion sizes.

# SAMPLE MENUS— PHASE THREE

### Day 1: The Basic Rice Diet

**To be enjoyed no more than one day per week without our medical supervision.**

| Breakfast: | 2 starches = 1 cup cooked steel-cut oats or oatmeal |
| | 1 fruit = 2 tablespoons dried cherries |
| | 1 fruit = ½ banana |

| Lunch: | 2 starches = ⅔ cup cooked brown basmati rice |
| | 1 fruit = 1 peach |
| | 1 fruit = 1 cup blueberries |

| Dinner: | 2 starches = ⅔ cup cooked brown basmati rice |
| | 1 fruit = 1 apple |
| | 1 fruit = 1 cup grapes, frozen |

### Days 2 to 5: The Lacto-Vegetarian Rice Diet

**To be enjoyed four days per week until weight and health goals are met. All foods in italics can be found in the recipe section, page 181.**

| Breakfast: | 1 starch = ½ cup grain cereal OR 1 slice toast |
| | 1 non-fat dairy = 1 cup non-fat soy, grain, or cow's milk (preferably organic) |
| | 1 fruit = 1 peach or 1 tablespoon all-fruit jam |

Lunch:
3 starches = 1½ cups of penne pasta

2 vegetables = 1 cup *Basic Tomato Sauce*

1 vegetable = ½ cup *Garlic Roasted Veggies*

1 fruit = 1 cup grapes

---

Dinner:
2 starches + 2 vegetables = *Red Bell Pepper with Orzo Stuffing*

1 starch + 1 vegetable = *Taco Salad*

1 fruit = 1 cup fresh berries

## Days 6 to 7: The Vegetarian Plus Rice Diet

**Same as the Lacto-Vegetarian Rice Diet + Fish, Lean Meat, or more Non-fat Dairy (an approximate 200 calorie addition); in Phase Three there are two days per week of enjoying these extra calories. (These do not need to be consecutive days.) Since maintenance is the goal at this point, if you are still losing next week you can enjoy three of these 1,200-calorie Vegetarian Plus days! All foods in italics can be found in the recipe section in Chapter 9.**

Breakfast:
2 starches = 1 cup cooked steel-cut oats or oat bran

½ fruit = 1 tablespoon raisins

½ fruit = ½ cup sliced strawberries

---

Lunch:
2 starches = ⅔ cup cooked Black Pearl rice

1½ starches = ½ cup *Black Beans 'n Garlic*

2 vegetables = 1 cup *Broccoli Rapini*

1 vegetable = *Baby Greens with Roasted Bell Peppers*

1 fruit = 1 pear

---

Dinner:
3 protein + 1 starch + 1 vegetable = *Seafood Gumbo*

2 vegetables = *Asparagus and Spinach Salad*

1½ starches + fruit = *Sweet Potato Pie*

# SERVING SIZES AND MORE

## SERVING SIZES

All menu suggestions in this chapter and later in the recipe section clearly indicate the number of servings you may find best to average for each meal. For instance, in the Basic Rice Diet, you will be eating 2 servings of starches and 2 servings of fruits for each breakfast, lunch, and dinner. During Phase Two, in the Lacto-Vegetarian Rice Diet, you will on average be eating 1 starch, 1 dairy, and 1 fruit for breakfast, and 3 starches, 3 vegetables, and 1 fruit for each lunch and dinner. But you don't need to memorize this information, nor is it carved in stone—just a reasonable way to spread these great calories through the day and minimize your setting yourself up for hunger. One of the most respected words of wisdom from those who have lost weight and kept it off is to eat breakfast, and in general, not skip meals.

## WHEN TO EAT

The average Ricer (while on the program) eats at 7:30 A.M., 12:30 P.M., and 5:30 P.M. If these times seem early to you and your family, personalize it to fit your life. Just remember that those who eat late have much more challenge with their weight than those who don't. Create a specific plan that you will commit to follow. You may modify this as you desire, but having your plan as specific as times to eat will only assist you in your mission. For example: "I will follow the Rice Diet eating no more than 1 extra fruit or vegetable per day, and no later than 7 P.M." Declaring your intentions, journalizing them so they are in black and white—possibly posted and visible on the refrigerator—will only help the home team.

# WATCHING YOUR FLUIDS AND FAT

We recommend drinking at least 40, but no more than 72 ounces of liquid per day. This is not a diet on which you should force fluids. Although weight loss is the goal in Phases One and Two, the small amounts of olive oil (1 to 2 teaspoons) in some recipes will not deter your progress. Also, you can always replace one starch in breakfast with one non-fat dairy (soy, grain, or cow's milk). They have virtually the same calories.

The table below clarifies the portion size in cups, ounces, tablespoons, and teaspoons for each food group, and the amount of calories and sodium in that serving for all the foods you will be eating.

| Food Group | 1 serving size in cup/ounces/teaspoon/tablespoon | Calories/ serving | Sodium |
|---|---|---|---|
| Starch—whole grains and starchy vegetables | ½ cup cooked | 80 | 2–5 mg |
| Starch—rice or beans | ⅓ cup cooked | 80 | 2–5 mg |
| Starch—bread | 1 slice | 80 | 2–160 mg |
| Vegetables | 1 cup raw ½ cup cooked | 25 | 5–20 mg |
| Fruits | 1 average piece of most whole fruits ½ banana 2 tablespoons raisins | 60 | 0–1 mg |

| Fruits (*cont.*) | ½ cup unsweetened juice or cooked fruit | 60 | 0–1 mg |
|---|---|---|---|
| Dairy | 1 cup non-fat soy, grain, or cow's milk or yogurt<br>½ cup dry curd cottage cheese | 90 | 126–150 mg |
| Protein | 1 ounce cooked fish<br>1 ounce cooked skinned poultry<br>1 ounce cooked lean meat<br>¼ cup cooked dried beans or peas | 55 | 51 mg |
| Fat | 1 teaspoon olive or canola oil<br>1 tablespoon sesame seeds or walnuts<br>1½ teaspoons seed or nut butter, or tahini<br>⅛ avocado | 45 | 0 |

As you get accustomed to the diet, you will probably be using this table as a reference. But soon, you will become familiar with the portion sizes and the number of servings, and you will be able to eyeball how much food you will be eating. For instance, a medium cereal bowl holds ¾ cup if you fill it almost to the top. So once you get comfortable with the serving sizes you can simply use the bowl to determine the right amount of food from each of the categories: starch, veggie, fruit, and protein or dairy. If you are ever hungry, it's a good tip to remember to eat your vegetables first; with less than half of the calories of any of the other food groups, it is always smartest to start eating the veggies, slowly and mindfully. This gives the nerves attached to your stomach time to tell your brain that you are not really that hungry. You can both slow down further and enjoy the higher calorie foods more and eat less of them.

# THE HEALTHY GROCERY LIST

Most people admit they would eat healthy meals if they were convenient. But it is up to you to take responsibility to make them convenient by ensuring these healthier foods are available in your refrigerator, cupboard, car, and office. The following staples and snacks make life easier and most are available at your local grocery store, the Rice Diet Store (you can order online at www.ricediet store.com or send for a catalog), or health food stores.*

## BEANS AND PEAS (LEGUMES)

• **Dried beans/peas**—any variety (they are less expensive when bought in bulk from food cooperatives). Bean Cuisine ◯ makes 8 soup kits that start with dried beans; no salt is included in the kit and each kit makes 14 tasty one-cup servings.

• **Frozen beans/peas**—no salt or fat added.

• **Canned beans**—no salt or fat added (Eden Organic is the best known no-salt-added brand) ◯.

• **Light Life Tempeh**—natural, unflavored has no sodium.

• **Nosoya Firm Tofu**—unflavored has no sodium.

• **Textured Vegetable Protein (TVP)** is available in bulk at many natural food stores ◯.

* Products on this healthy list that are available at the Rice Diet Store are marked with a ◯.

# BEVERAGES

The average American's beverage is loaded with caffeine, sodium, fat, sugar, and/or artificial sweeteners. All of these can be potentially harmful. Even the decaffeinated beverages have some potentially adverse effects. Decaffeinated coffee and/or tea have been shown to aggravate hernias and inhibit the absorption of iron from 39 to 87 percent respectively. If you really want some decaffeinated coffee, look for "naturally decaffeinated" coffee. But try some healthier alternatives, such as my personal favorite, Orzo ☼ (an Italian coffee substitute made from roasted barley), or Decopa ☼, which is roasted dahlia root. However, there are many other healthy beverage choices:

• **Water, bottled spring water, or distilled seltzer water**—salt-free varieties; good when mixed with 100 percent fruit juices.

• **Herbal teas, decaffeinated and unsweetened, preferably;** green tea contains high amounts of health promoting antioxidants—good quality brands include Harney & Sons, Tazo, and the Republic of Tea. If you don't care for the taste of green tea straight, mixing it with flavorful fruity blends (like Tazo's Passion) masks the green tea's rather bland flavor, and it is incredible iced.

• **Fruit juices unsweetened;** check ingredients to confirm fruit juice only or fruit juice and seltzer water blends.

• **Vegetable juices** unsalted are great if you add lemon, lime, or other salt- and fat-free condiments, such as horseradish and low-sodium Worcestershire sauce.

• **Milk: soy and grain milks, skim, ½ percent, and 1 percent are recommended** in this order. Soy and grain milks have some advantages over cow's milk. When compared to 2 percent cow's milk, Edensoy Extra Original provides more protein and plant-based estrogens called isoflavones. Isoflavones, especially genistein, are be-

> # REMEMBER TO DRINK BETWEEN 40 AND 72 OUNCES OF FLUID PER DAY!

ing studied for their reported ability to reduce the risk of cancer. Researchers currently suggest 50 milligrams of isoflavones each day for the possible prevention of cancer. Soymilk is an excellent replacement for cow milk, with less saturated fat, more protein, and provides 20 milligrams of soy isoflavones per cup.

# BREADS AND CRACKERS

Most people with overeating problems find that breads and crackers trigger their desire for eating too much, thus creating weight gain. And, traditionally, breads or starchy snacks have more fat. However, if you can eat a slice of bread without triggering cravings, you can have a slice of bread (preferably whole grain without hydrogenated fats) as one starch. In addition, almost all of these commercially available products, except for those made at a health-oriented bakery, will contain partially hydrogenated fat, which raises blood cholesterol and increases the risk of heart disease. The following choices can be found without any sodium or saturated fat–rich ingredients.

• **Corn tortillas** can easily be found containing only corn, lime, and water

• **Galilee Splendor Bible Bread with Honey** ☼

• **Bremner Crackers**—unsalted ☼

- **Edward and Sons Sesame Unsalted Rice Snaps** ☼

- **Hol-grain Brown Rice Cracker**—no-salt-added ☼

- **Old London Sesame and Whole Grain Melba Toasts**—no-salt-added varieties ☼

- **Matzos**—no-salt-added variety

- **Whole Wheat Pita Bread** (see Appendix for ordering Toufayan no-salt-added variety)

- **Rice Cakes**—no-fat and no-salt-added varieties (Koyo Millet ☼ has more flavor than regular rice cakes)

- **Ezekiel 4:9 bread,** low sodium, is available in the freezer section of natural foods groceries. It has 80 calories per slice and no sodium. It is best toasted.

# COLD CEREALS

Most cereals contain partially hydrogenated fats and 200 to 300 milligrams of sodium. The following have no added fat or sodium and 6 grams or less of added sugar or sucrose making them superior choices to the majority of cereals sold in chain grocery stores.

- **Puffed Rice and Wheat**

- **Raisin Squares**

- **Shredded Wheat**

The following cereals are found in a growing number of health food sections in the larger chain grocery stores. Of course, health food cooperatives or stores would have the largest selection.

- **Grainfield's cereals**

- **Health Valley's cereals**

- **Most New Morning cereals**
- **Kashi Cereals**
- **Nature's Path Granola** ○

# HOT CEREALS

Excellent choices for hot cereals are:

- **Buckwheat groats** (also known as kasha) ○
- **Cream of Rice** (or Rice and Shine) ○
- **Cream of Wheat**—White or Whole Wheat (or Cream of Rye) ○
- **Grits** ○
- **Hodgens Mill Multigrain Cereal** ○
- **Kashi**—a brand name for a 7-grain and sesame mixed cereal
- **Oats:** Oat groats, steel-cut oats, oat bran, oatmeal ○
- **Wheat and Rye Farina** (Farina is the same as cream of wheat) ○

Most health food stores have numerous other hot and cold cereals. Take care to read the ingredients and choose one without added sodium or fat; the nutritional analysis should read no more than 2 grams of fat, 10 milligrams of sodium, 6 grams of added sugar, and at least 2 grams of fiber.

# WHOLE GRAINS

The ultimate cereal is the whole grain itself before it has been puffed, flaked, or processed in any way. Most refined products have half the fiber content and significantly fewer nutrients than the original whole grain. The following can be found at most health food stores and a growing number of chain groceries. (These types of grains should be the foundation of starches in your diet.)

• **Amaranth**—South American grain offering a nice thickener to soups, or can be popped like miniature popcorn to add crunch to salads, high in protein and vitamin E

• **Barley**—hulled, pearled, flaked, or barley flour

• **Kasha** (roasted buckwheat groats)

• **Millet**—toasting millet for 10 minutes before boiling it improves the flavor and texture dramatically

• **Oat groats, or Irish (steel-cut) oats**

• **Pasta, couscous, and fregole** are usually processed wheat products, the latter two are small versions ☼

• **Polenta** (finely to coarsely ground corn; the 5-minute variety comes without salt) ☼

• **Popcorn**—air-popped or microwave from scratch, no oil or salt ☼

• **Quinoa**—South American grain that is relatively new to the U.S.; it has a great crunch and mouth feel ☼

• **Rice**—brown, wild, basmati, Black Pearl, or any type that does not contain added fat and sodium ☼

• **Rye berries**—flakes or flour

• **Wheat berries, bulgur (cracked wheat)** ☼**, germ and bran**— the latter two are fractions of the former whole

# CONDIMENTS

The ultimate condiments to substitute for the traditional salt and fat laden ones are herbs, lemon, lime, and the many varieties of herbed vinegars. But the following condiments are convenient and available at the Rice Diet Store and some grocery stores.

- **Balsamic vinegar** ☼

- **Conserves or fruit only jams/jellies/fruit spreads** ☼

- **Cherchies no-salt herb seasoning mixes** ☼

- **Frontier no salt seasoning mixes**—many varieties ☼

- **Diet Zing low-sodium hot sauce** ☼

- **Enrico's No Salt or Desert Pepper Peach Mango Salsa** ☼

- **Heinz or Hunt's no-salt-added ketchup** ☼

- **Mr. Spice sauces**—many to choose from, all no salt/no fat added ☼

- **Molasses, honey, brown sugar, and anything ending in "ose"** should be limited due to empty calories. Molasses is the only sweetener with any significant nutritional value.

- **Paul Prudhomme's Magic seasoning,** no-salt-added variety ☼

- **Angostura Worcestershire sauce,** low-sodium variety ☼

- **The Ginger People** have a number of condiments with no salt added: **Sweet Ginger Chili** and the **Sushi Ginger** are both excellent but the sugar content is higher ☼

# CONVENIENCE FOODS

As you might have noticed, many products advertise low or no fat, sodium, or sugar, but rarely are they low in all three! The following convenience foods are free or very low in all of these concerns. Remember to use a little imagination in preparing convenience foods that have no added salt or fat. For instance, fresh squeezed lemon and lime and no-salt condiments, such as mustard and horseradish, can instantly jazz up many low-sodium convenience foods.

• **Spaghetti sauce** no-salt-added, produced by **Roselli's** ○ or **Walnut Acres**

• **Frozen vegetables** for quick stir fries

• **Bearitos Vegetarian Refried Beans,** no-salt-added ○

• **Health Valley,** no-salt-added products, especially the Vegetarian Chili ○

• **Marco Polo Ajvar** ○—a mild or hot sauce of peppers, eggplant, and garlic is an excellent pasta, rice, potato, or veggie topping and can even be used as a pizza sauce on pita pizza

• **Muir Glen** or **Eden Tomato Sauces,** no-salt-added ○

# DAIRY PRODUCTS

All dairy products are fairly high in sodium and protein, averaging 126 milligrams of sodium and 8 grams of protein per cup of skim milk. The following products are your lowest fat and sodium choices:

• **Low-sodium cottage cheese** if less than 65 milligrams sodium

• **Nonfat plain yogurt with active yogurt cultures** (Stonyfield Farm is best).

• **Skim milk**

• **Non-dairy alternatives** include soy milk (Edensoy or WestSoy), soy yogurt (Whole Soy Creamy Cultured Soy), and almond and grain milk.

# DETERMINING YOUR GOALS

Now let's understand why we weigh what we weigh. We require a certain number of calories per pound to maintain our weight. This number is mainly dependent on our muscle mass and decreases as we get older, because our muscle mass usually decreases as we get older unless we're committed to serious bodybuilding. The number of calories used per pound is slightly higher for men than for women because men usually have more muscle mass than women at any given weight. The number of calories we use per pound also varies depending on our activity level.

## HOW MUCH SHOULD I WEIGH? DETERMINING YOUR BMI

In order to establish your weight loss goals, you first need to figure out your Body Mass Index (BMI), the simplest and best common measure of weight for height. BMI is calculated by dividing a person's weight (in kilograms) by the square of his height (in meters). Since Americans still use the English system, the formula for calculating BMI is as follows:

$$\text{BMI} = \frac{703 \times \text{weight in pounds}}{\text{height in inches} \times \text{height in inches}}$$

Or, you can simply consult the chart on page 51.

| BMI (kg/m²) | 19 | 20 | 21 | 22 | 23 | 24 | 25 | 26 | 27 | 28 | 29 | 30 | 35 | 40 |
|---|---|---|---|---|---|---|---|---|---|---|---|---|---|---|
| Height (in.) | Weight (lbs.) | | | | | | | | | | | | | |
| 58 | 91 | 96 | 100 | 105 | 110 | 115 | 119 | 124 | 129 | 134 | 138 | 143 | 167 | 191 |
| 59 | 94 | 99 | 104 | 109 | 114 | 119 | 124 | 128 | 133 | 138 | 143 | 148 | 173 | 198 |
| 60 | 97 | 102 | 107 | 112 | 118 | 123 | 128 | 133 | 138 | 143 | 148 | 153 | 179 | 204 |
| 61 | 100 | 106 | 111 | 116 | 122 | 127 | 132 | 137 | 143 | 148 | 153 | 158 | 185 | 211 |
| 62 | 104 | 109 | 115 | 120 | 126 | 131 | 136 | 142 | 147 | 153 | 158 | 164 | 191 | 218 |
| 63 | 107 | 113 | 118 | 124 | 130 | 135 | 141 | 146 | 152 | 158 | 163 | 169 | 197 | 225 |
| 64 | 110 | 116 | 122 | 128 | 134 | 140 | 145 | 151 | 157 | 163 | 169 | 174 | 204 | 232 |
| 65 | 114 | 120 | 126 | 132 | 138 | 144 | 150 | 156 | 162 | 168 | 174 | 180 | 210 | 240 |
| 66 | 118 | 124 | 130 | 136 | 142 | 148 | 155 | 161 | 167 | 173 | 179 | 186 | 216 | 247 |
| 67 | 121 | 127 | 134 | 140 | 146 | 153 | 159 | 166 | 172 | 178 | 185 | 191 | 223 | 255 |
| 68 | 125 | 131 | 138 | 144 | 151 | 158 | 164 | 171 | 177 | 184 | 190 | 197 | 230 | 262 |
| 69 | 128 | 135 | 142 | 149 | 155 | 162 | 169 | 176 | 182 | 189 | 196 | 203 | 236 | 270 |
| 70 | 132 | 139 | 146 | 153 | 160 | 167 | 174 | 181 | 188 | 195 | 202 | 207 | 243 | 278 |
| 71 | 136 | 143 | 150 | 157 | 165 | 172 | 179 | 186 | 193 | 200 | 208 | 215 | 250 | 286 |
| 72 | 140 | 147 | 154 | 162 | 169 | 177 | 184 | 191 | 199 | 206 | 213 | 221 | 258 | 294 |
| 73 | 144 | 151 | 159 | 166 | 174 | 182 | 189 | 197 | 204 | 212 | 219 | 227 | 265 | 302 |
| 74 | 148 | 155 | 163 | 171 | 179 | 186 | 194 | 202 | 210 | 218 | 225 | 233 | 272 | 311 |
| 75 | 152 | 160 | 168 | 176 | 184 | 192 | 200 | 208 | 216 | 224 | 232 | 240 | 279 | 319 |
| 76 | 156 | 164 | 172 | 180 | 189 | 197 | 205 | 213 | 221 | 230 | 238 | 246 | 287 | 328 |

**Body weight in pounds according to height and body mass index.**

Most authorities consider a BMI less than 25 to be healthy; above 25, the person is considered overweight; above 30, obese. Optimally, your BMI should be less than 23. Indeed, the literature clearly shows that the leaner you are, the longer you'll live.

# WHAT IS MY NORMAL WEIGHT?

Calculating your BMI gives you a good understanding of what a healthy weight would be for you. At the Rice Diet Program, in addition to BMI, we also ask how much a person weighed at age eighteen. Most people will give you a number within 10 pounds of what would be their healthiest weight. Even most people who were overweight at age eighteen would give their eyeteeth to weigh what they did when they were eighteen. We pick eighteen because most people do not grow taller after eighteen so they don't add any bone, and very few add any muscle. So, that leaves fat, which we don't need.

So once you have this information, you should have a fairly good idea of what your optimal weight is. Now it's up to you to decide what you want to weigh and how much you need to lose to achieve that goal.

# HOW MUCH CAN I EXPECT TO LOSE? USING THE ROSATI METHOD

The Rosati method of helping you to determine a realistic weight loss strategy is simple. It starts with the premise that it takes 10 calo-

ries per pound to maintain your weight. Sure this is an approxima-
tion since the number depends on your sex, activity, and so on, but
it's so easy to multiply by ten and it's close enough.

For example, if you weigh 150 pounds, it takes about 1,500 calories to maintain your weight. If you weigh 200 pounds, it takes 2,000
calories, 250 pounds 2,500 calories, and so on. Most of these calories
are used to heat our bodies. Additional calories are needed if we exercise regularly. As a general rule, walking uses about 100 calories
per mile. Again, this depends on your weight and sex and how fast
you are going, but it's close enough.

So if you weigh 150 pounds and walk for an hour a day (say
3 miles) you need about 1,800 calories to maintain your weight:
1,500 + 300. If you weigh 250 pounds, you need about 2,800 calories
to maintain your weight with the one-hour walk per day. These are
probably underestimates of the number of calories needed, but you
can always add calories if you get too thin!

Now, let's see how to use this knowledge to figure out a weight
loss program. To keep it simple let's forget about the effects of exercise for a minute. Exercise does help you to lose weight but the effect is small compared with limiting calories. (We shall see later that
exercise is very important in keeping weight off.)

Suppose you weigh 230 pounds and want to weigh 170 pounds.
At 230, it takes about 2,300 calories to maintain your weight. You
could just reduce your caloric intake to 1,700 and wait. There are
about 3,500 to 3,600 calories in a pound of fat. With 600 calories less
intake per day you'd lose a little over a pound a week. It would take
about a year to get to 170 pounds. It would probably take longer
since the more you lose, the fewer calories you need to maintain
your weight and the less the deficit per day.

If you weigh 230 and eat 800 calories per day, you would have a
1,500 calorie per day deficit (2,300 - 800 = 1,500) and you would lose
about a half a pound a day. If you added in a one-hour walk, you
would have a 1,800 deficit, and it would take you about 3 to 4 months
to get to 170 pounds.

An important thing to note from these examples is that the difference between weighing 170 pounds and 230 pounds is only 600 calories per day for a year. Six hundred calories a day makes the difference between weighing 170 or weighing 110 or between weighing 280 or 220. Six hundred calories is an hour's walk and a handful of peanuts. Most of us are not overweight because we are eating horribly wrong but because we are making a small error every day.

One woman came to us weighing 140 pounds. She wanted to weigh 110. Twenty pounds is two Cokes a day. That was it. The two Cokes she was drinking each day equaled 20 pounds of excessive weight at the end of the year. Those two Cokes were the difference between her weighing 140 and 112 because she was drinking them every day. She could have kept drinking the Cokes and walked an hour a day and she would also have weighed about 112 pounds a year later. Of course, she would have to take that hour walk every day.

Another man came to us weighing 120 pounds more than he desired. He said he was a gourmet cook and knew he wasn't eating that much. He didn't use much fat or oil in his cooking. We asked if he ate between meals. "No," he didn't. Did he drink? "Maybe one or two drinks a year," he responded. We were stymied. What was he doing to cause his overweight? It still wasn't clear.

In talking with the man further, he mentioned in passing that he was a wine collector. "What do you do with all that wine," I asked, thinking about his comment that he only had one or two drinks a year. "Oh, I drink at least a bottle a day," the man answered. He obviously didn't consider drinking wine to be "drinking." Wine was food to him. Well, there was 80 of the 120 pounds! Alcohol is calories: about 100 calories per ounce for liquor or three ounces of wine. The man then went on to remember the appetizers he usually had with a glass of white or sparkling wine before dinner—the other 40 pounds. By drinking a bottle of wine each day and adding a few appetizers he was consistently taking in 1,200 calories more than he needed.

# ARE YOU READY?

Although eating the foods on the Rice Diet is enjoyable and easy, making the multidimensional commitment to transform your life can often feel intimidating and challenging. You have to be open to making such a change in your life, believe in your own power to make such changes, and also trust that you can and will learn to eat in this new way. As T.C. said, "I came to the Rice Diet Program one year and four months ago weighing 468 pounds. Since then, I have lost 220 pounds. But more than just losing the weight, I have gained the knowledge of how to live my life without 'dieting' ever again. The Rice Diet Program is more than just a diet program; it has saved my life. I now understand the true nature of foods, especially the flavor-enhancing, binge-producing response that salt has on my body. I believe many would say they don't want to change much in their lives, they just want to lose weight. They miss the power and potential of the Rice Diet. I was ready before I came here to make big changes and I made the right choice. When I came here, this felt like my last chance. I was willing to sell my business, dissolve relationships, and literally move my life to a place where I knew no one and nothing. Being ready is essential; however, the Rice Diet Program welcomes you offering the emotional healing and support that you need for such a life-changing transformation."

T.C. embraced the diet and, more important, a new *dieta* for the life-transforming results she dreamed were possible in her life. Are you ready to make the choice to reach and maintain your desired weight in a new way that will inspire you to feel better, think more clearly, feel physically stronger and more energetic? Are you ready to either prevent disease from insinuating itself in your body or reverse health conditions that have already crept up on you? Are you truly ready to change your life? If you can answer yes to even one of these changes, then you are indeed ready. Remember, you will not feel isolated or alone as you do this program. We have many suggestions for you to find support, encouragement, and comfort at all stages of this experience in the upcoming chapters—so hold on for the ride of your life!

# CHAPTER THREE

# WILL I FEEL HUNGRY? AND OTHER QUESTIONS ABOUT THE RICE DIET

*We cannot solve problems with the same level of consciousness that created them.*

—ALBERT EINSTEIN

W e've assembled here all the most commonly asked questions about the Rice Diet. Here you will learn more about how it feels to be on the Rice Diet, and all the little questions that arise along the way.

## Will I feel hungry?

Although the calories in Phase One are significantly less than we usually average, most people say they don't experience hunger. As one woman said, "I was shocked. I couldn't believe that one thousand calories a day would be enough. I was afraid that I would start bingeing at night, but amazingly I didn't feel hungry at all. I also slept like a baby!"

Real hunger is your stomach/body telling your brain that you need nourishment. But when most people say they are hungry they are describing more a state of mind or an emotional feeling rather than true physiological hunger. As one man explained, "When I first started the Rice Diet I always thought I was hungry. But when I began to really think about it, I realized it wasn't hunger I was feeling but anxiety about being able to feel full. The more I became conscious of what I was eating, the more slowly I ate. I realized I did feel full after every meal and I never had cravings between meals. It was so liberating!" On the Rice Diet, by eating whole foods, you will give yourself time to realize you're satiated and thereby win the race with the signal from your stomach to your brain in time to prevent overeating, snacking, or bingeing.

## How does the Rice Diet detox the body?

The other magical aspect of the Rice Diet is that it is like a fast in that you are cleansed not only of excessive sodium, but of other unnatural substances or amounts that you may have previously consumed, especially when you do one day a week of the Basic Rice Diet. This is probably an impossible aspect to actually quantify or prove but many signs of detoxification occur. For example, many come to the program with a caffeine habit that they do not even recognize. Even those participants with a two-cup-a-day habit of coffee or soda may experience headaches for their first few days on the program. You can eliminate or minimize this symptom by gradually drinking less and less coffee, tea, or soda for a week until you are off it. You can take headache medication while needed or tough it out. But, otherwise, most people describe only positive responses, including an almost immediate improvement in sleep pattern, allergies, arthritis-like joint stiffness, energy level (after the first week your energy will markedly increase), attitude, and perspective on life in general.

## Why rice?

One of the first questions people often ask us as they contemplate doing the Rice Diet is, "Do I only eat rice?" The answer is no.

When Dr. Walter Kempner first developed the Rice Diet, he designed it to treat high blood pressure and kidney disease. Although we cannot be 100 percent certain why Dr. Kempner selected rice, we believe it was because of two qualities: (1) it is a grain and so contains very little naturally occurring sodium, and (2) most of the world's people who don't suffer from chronic diseases enjoy this highly nutritious, easy-to-grow staple. Indeed, many people consume rice more than any food in their diet. Dr. Kempner's answer was, "It's not what's in the rice, it's what's not in the rice." It turns out that rice contains a fairly complete protein. Now, we encourage people to eat other grains as well, the more complex or "whole" the better. Oatmeal, steel-cut oats, and oat bran are three breakfast favorites. In addition, participants also enjoy barley, kamut, and quinoa.

## Why do I only eat one day of the Basic Rice Diet?

You eat only one day of the Basic Rice Diet because it is so low in sodium it should not be eaten day after day without daily, experienced medical supervision. At the Rice Diet Program we call the

Basic Rice Diet "rice and fruit," even though it actually includes all grains. Your one day of the Basic Rice Diet has an important role to play in changing your eating behavior to a healthier one.

First, eating the Basic Rice Diet for a day lets us appreciate how wonderful a carrot or a salad or a baked potato really tastes. This realization is pivotal. All of us have the tendency to seek or long for something we don't have because we fail to appreciate what we do have. No matter what we possess—material things, good health, a loving relationship, a supportive family, professional success—we get caught in the "I'm-bored-with-what-I-have" trap and we end up associating what we have with being "not enough," and blaming feeling bored on "it." However, when we eat rice and fruit for one day each week something magical happens: we appreciate what we have (i.e., other food choices the rest of the week). This experience and awareness enables us to appreciate all that we have in our lives—not just rice and fruit and veggies and some freshly cooked, delicious, savory fish, but all that we are blessed with in our lives. Dr. Rosati realized this, too. As he tells the Ricers, "I never could understand how I could ever be bored. I am intelligent. I have many interests. How can I be bored? I finally realized I am only bored when I fail to appreciate what I have. Now, in the evening, when I'm bored, I go upstairs and look at my son sleeping. And, I'm not bored."

And, second, if you can eat the Basic Rice Diet one day a week, you're cured from being powerless over food. Eating the Basic Rice Diet one day a week enables you to become focused and mindful of what you are thinking, feeling, and doing. On one of my rice and fruit days, I (Kitty) found myself standing in a coffee shop eating a brownie. I wasn't sure how I got there, but I realized three-fourths of the way through the brownie that someone had hurt my feelings, and that I was comforting myself with my "drug" of choice. Although I had been attending eating disorder workshops for years as a Registered Dietitian, I had no idea that I ever ate for emotional reasons. All of us, regardless of our weight or health, eat for emotional reasons. When you truly begin to change your *dieta*, detox with a whole foods diet, educate yourself on the nutritional value of your food selections, and seek the inner healing we explore further in Chapter 5, you will naturally become conscious of why you eat for emotional reasons and how to heal this response. Eating rice and fruit one day a week allows your sense of your own power to surface—the power to eat rice and fruit only. You have created a new habit—to eat wisely and well. And when eating this way is reinforced by losing weight, this new habit is reinforced again.

## Why is the Rice Diet a Low-Sodium Diet and What Does This Mean?

Low sodium is good for you because it minimizes your over-eating triggers. Salt, like refined sugar, is an appetite stimulant. Without added salt you will eat less. If you've been on the Rice Diet, you know that you don't feel hungry almost after the first meal. This absence of hunger occurs no matter how good the food is. If you've never been on the Rice Diet, you'll just have to take our word for it.

Of course, there are many other health benefits from lowering your sodium intake, including the resulting reduction in blood pressure, joint pain, diabetes complications, and risks of numerous other diseases, including congestive heart failure, osteoporosis, and stomach cancer. See Chapter 8 for other medical advantages of a low-sodium diet.

Occasionally using cheese as a condiment is okay. If you eat a lot of it habitually, it isn't. If you choose to be very low sodium, you are better off avoiding cheese. We challenge our heart patients (who want to do all they can naturally to reverse their disease) to think of cheese and meat, other than fish, in the historical sense!

## What about sweets?

When most people say sweets, they mean chocolate, candy bars, cake, or cookies. These foods may taste sweet because they have sugar in them, but they are primarily fat. The obvious best alternative is the freshest, ripest organically grown fruit; buy them at the farmers' market from the grower who picked them that morning.

## Can I eat bread?

The majority of the world who are much thinner than those living in industrialized nations eat more bread than we do. The main difference is that their bread is not as processed. If you are eating whole-grain bread that you can see is filled with half-split grains and has a heavy weight, then you are much safer than if it's light, white, and fluffy. Good whole grain, homemade breads usually don't have significant amounts of undesirable fats in them. Bread can usually be found without added salt, but not in all grocery stores. The Tuscan bread recipe in this book is delicious; this region of Italy traditionally makes bread without salt. It's supposed to be eaten with food and it's great. See page 45 for Ezekiel 4:9 and other good choices in the Healthy Grocery List.

## Should I be concerned about losing muscle during rapid weight loss?

It is true that some muscle is lost during weight loss, but this muscle is quickly restored with exercise. Your body is very smart about conserving more important muscles; for instance, your body would use skeletal muscle rather than heart muscle if it needed more energy. Your body may lose a little muscle, but you can do a lot more exercise with the weight loss than before you lost the weight, thus muscle mass will be up before any loss is even noticed.

## The Rice Diet seems low in protein; is that dangerous?

The Rice Diet has been helping people heal and optimize their health naturally for over sixty-five years. As Dr. Kempner showed years ago, we need much less protein than we think. The Rice Diet has more than sufficient protein so don't worry. We have not seen protein deficiencies develop while a patient is here losing weight on the Rice Diet Program. (See page 80 for the story of C., who not only lost weight on the Rice Diet but continued to develop his muscle mass and strength through weight lifting.)

## How much water do I need to drink?

Since the Rice Diet is so low in sodium, you do not need to drink a lot of fluids. Your total fluid intake should be about 40 to 72 ounces a day, which is equivalent to 5 to 9 glasses a day. If you are exercising more than one hour each day or if the weather is unusually hot, then you may increase your water intake to about 9 to 10 glasses a day and be sure you are including dairy and regular bread or cereal in your diet daily, or an extra 200 milligrams of sodium as desired.

## What about coffee and caffeinated drinks?

You can also drink decaffeinated soda, tea, and coffee, and fruit juice. We recommend that you stay away from diet sodas and coffee for a couple of reasons: (1) caffeine is a stimulant and may interfere with the inner calm you are achieving on the Rice Diet and in your life and (2) the additives in soda are harmful to your health. For example, the dietary phosphate found in high amounts in sodas—and meat—causes an increase in calcium loss, which is not a good thing for women (and men) avoiding osteoporosis.

## Can I have any alcohol on the Rice Diet?

We are of two minds when it comes to alcohol: (1) Alcohol can easily be used in excess so don't drink and (2) Alcohol is derived from either a grain, vegetable, or fruit and this is a grain, vegetable, and fruit diet.

In other words, if you don't drink don't start. The possible health benefits of alcohol are far outweighed by the risk of abuse. If you do drink, studies have shown that there may be some health benefits to moderate drinking, especially red wine (due to resveratrol, an antioxidant and anticancer agent). Alcohol does contain 7 kcal/g. This translates roughly into 100 kcal for three ounces of wine or one ounce of hard liquor. You have to account for the calories. If you daily added two glasses (3-ounce glasses please) of wine to your present diet and changed nothing else (vis-à-vis caloric intake or output), you would gain about 20 pounds in a year. Also, remember that alcohol can reduce your self-control and make it more challenging for you to prioritize your eating plan. It seems to me that the safest thing to do, if you do drink, is to drink with your meal and not before or after meals. Obviously, it would be best to avoid alcohol until Phase Three, then do so consciously by journalizing and taking notes.

## Can I use herbs and spices?

It may seem obvious when you are on a low-sodium diet but just in case: don't add salt to your food. Watch your spices as well. Herbs and spices will enhance not only the flavor of various foods but also your enjoyment of them. For example, topping your oatmeal with cinnamon can be a wonderful treat. But there is one risk of using spices: you might eat more. So use them wisely. (You will learn much more about trying and adding herbs and spices to your foods in Chapter 6.)

## What about using sauces and dressings on food?

Ready-made condiments, sauces, and marinades are popular in our fast-paced world, and the low-sodium versions are getting tastier and easier to find. If they taste a bit flat, use your imagination and jazz them up with fresh lemons, limes, horseradish, wasabi, fresh and dried herbs, dried chili peppers, and chipotle peppers (smoked jalapeños), or a variety of vinegars, mustards, and ketchup. The Rice Diet Store sells and ships the best selection of salt-free products we have seen anywhere, from hot sauces, stir fry sauces, marinades, and dressings, to the best balsamic vinegars and extra virgin olive oils we've tasted.

## What if I want more sodium?

Optimally your sodium intake should be between 500 and 1,000 milligrams of sodium per day. It is impossible to get to 1,000 milligrams without adding processed foods or salt. At home, we never add salt to our food, but we do use sun-dried tomatoes and other flavorful no-salt-added ingredients, whereas anchovies, olives, and cheese are used more sparingly. Chopped sun-dried tomatoes give a salty hit to your taste buds, but don't really contain much sodium (read the label to be sure salt has not been added; see Appendix A to order no-salt-added type). Four pieces of sun-dried tomatoes contain only 20 milligrams of sodium in 60 calories. Anchovies, olives, and cheese are processed with salt but, if we are conscious, a little bit can go a long way. Two anchovies contain 143 milligrams of sodium in 8 calories, 5 kalamata olives contain 200 milligrams of sodium in 45 calories, and 1 tablespoon of grated Parmesan cheese contains 93 milligrams of sodium in 23 calories. Our concern with these latter food additions is that they are often foods that participants say they need to avoid until their health and weight goals have been achieved. So when entering these "slippery slopes" do so with a journal in hand and weigh daily, to assess weekly whether these additions are what you are ready to include in your *dieta* at this time.

## Can I add an artificial sweetener to my decaf tea or coffee?

At every meal you may have either 1 packet of sugar, Sweet 'N Low, Equal, Splenda, 1 teaspoon of honey, or 1 teaspoon of maple syrup. Since a teaspoon of any natural sweetner has approximately 16 calories, limiting them to 1 teaspoon per day is optimal. We highly recommend that you eliminate artificial sweeteners. Artificial sweeteners have an intense flavor that gives the taste buds an amazing hit and limits your ability to taste real food. They also can make nonedible foods edible. One morning we were saying hello to one of our favorite patients and noticed that her grapefruit looked like it had been snowed upon. The grapefruit plate was surrounded by packets of Splenda. When we asked her why she was using so much sweetener, she responded that the grapefruit was sour. Then why was she eating it? We suggested she might prefer a fruit that was perfectly ripe and naturally sweet.

When Ricers want to sweeten a steel-cut oat breakfast, a small quantity of raisins and cinnamon are the ultimate!

## INSPIRATIONAL CORNER

F.N., a woman in her early fifties, said this about her experience on the Rice Diet Program: "I came to the Rice House weighing 332 pounds, and I couldn't walk from my car to the Rice House. I now weigh 198 pounds and I am committed to my goals. I had tried many diets before but always failed. I had learned the eating part but never learned the other parts of the diet. Now I exercise regularly. At first all I could do was walk a few steps and sit down. That's how I started. Now I can walk the trail at a brisk pace! I can't tell you how this diet has changed my life. I am getting out more, and I am finally taking care of myself. Sometimes it is exhausting to always be thinking about food, but I know that once I reach my goals, then doing [Phase Three] won't require as much energy. But the more days I live this [dieta], the easier and more normal it feels."

## CHAPTER FOUR

# BECOMING A MINDFUL EATER BEGINS WITH NUTRITION

*He who distinguishes the true savor of food can never be a glutton; he who does not cannot be otherwise.*

—HENRY DAVID THOREAU

"*B*ut *I just like to eat.*" We hear this all the time. Unfortunately, it's almost never true. Many people think of themselves as food lovers, but their actions speak louder than their words: they eat while they are talking; they eat while watching television; they eat standing up or while driving in their car. They eat so quickly and unconsciously that there is no way they can possibly be enjoying the food. If we really loved food, we would eat slowly, pay more attention to it, and eat it with reverence. If we liked to eat, we would use less or no salt so that we could taste the food itself.

Often when people stop and think about the food they're eating, they realize they're truly tasting it for the first time. When we began working with Dr. Kempner, one of the participants explained that he thought he could do okay without any added salt—except with corn on the cob. Corn on the cob demanded butter and salt. One day, he happened to encounter some corn on the cob without butter or salt. It was surprisingly delicious, sweet, and tender. But the next time he tried corn on the cob without butter or salt, it was awful, tough, and tasteless, and should have been fed to the pigs. He had learned something important: With butter and salt, he had never been able to tell the difference between fresh corn and old corn that sat in a grocery store for a week after traveling on a truck for a week before that. He had never known the difference because all he had been tasting was the butter and salt, not the corn underneath.

Our point? We are asking you to eat certain foods, not just because they are healthful and will help you lose weight, but because we want you to experience food and eating as a mindful activity that is worth your attention. We want you to be present so that you are able to truly enjoy real food worthy of your vessel.

# BECOMING MINDFUL

Being mindful is essential to make the Rice Diet work for you. By "being mindful" we mean thinking about what you're experiencing as you're experiencing it, being aware of your thoughts, your feelings, and your five senses. The more mindful and aware you are of yourself and the world around you, the more able you are to experience life instead of floating through it anesthetized. Who wants to wake up twenty years later to realize that your life has passed you by, you weigh 300 pounds, and your heart is about to explode?

The Rice Diet offers you a number of ways to become mindful, and becoming a mindful eater is just one of them. At the Rice House we offer a weekly or periodic Meditative Lunch in which we sit in silence as we eat. The lunch begins with remembering silently that this food is a gift and that when we treat it with respect, it will nourish us and promote health. This remembering can be in the form of a grace, which can be as informal as stating out loud our gratefulness for the food before us, or as formal as the reading of Thich Nhat Hanh's "Five Contemplations" (see box on page 70). We chew each bite fully before taking another, putting down our utensils between bites. At five to ten minute intervals, a harmonic bell sounds, signaling us to put down our fork and reflect upon what we are eating. We can either look at nothing or exchange smiles with our table mates, but we don't speak. We take this time to think about what we are eating, to taste the flavors, feel the texture of the foods, and become truly mindful of eating as an activity.

## THE FIVE CONTEMPLATIONS

This food is the gift of the whole universe: the earth, the sky and much hard work.

May we live mindfully so as to be worthy to receive it.

May we transform our unskillful states of mind and learn to eat with moderation.

May we take only foods that nourish us and prevent illness.

We accept this food in order to realize the path of understanding and love.

*Thich Nhat Hanh*

This may seem a little outlandish to do at home. But try it—even for just ten minutes. Put away your newspaper. Turn off the television or radio. Sit down and stop talking. Eat slowly. Chew each morsel fully and completely, taking in the texture, the smell, and the taste of the food. Smile to your companions. You will become grateful and aware. You will become sensitive and alert. You will become a mindful eater.

Here's another example or path used by many support groups in their quest to become mindful eaters. A group of people sit in a circle. They are given three raisins. One at a time, each person smells the raisin, feels it, observes its crinkly edges, and admires it. Each person thinks about how the raisin became a raisin: what was its journey from a grape? Then it's time to taste the raisin. Each person puts one in his or her mouth, feels its tactile sensation on the tongue, and takes in its succulent taste. After chewing it thoroughly, he swallows it. Now it's time to do the same with the next raisin.

Becoming mindful is about becoming grateful for the food we

are eating, and the raisin exercise, though simple, is a powerful way to focus on food in all its glory. One woman described this as "better than a gallon of Ben & Jerry's." Another participant said, "The best raisin I ever tasted was the first one I ate in this way."

So on your way to full mindfulness, take this short step and educate yourself about nutrition. We are certain that when you know about the foods you are eating, you automatically make better choices, which in turn enables you to take better care of yourself.

Again, doing the Rice Diet Program is not simply a matter of eating the foods prescribed and following directions, it's about becoming aware of why you eat the foods suggested. You may think that worrying about the nutritional content of food is better left to dietitians and physicians. Nothing could be further from the truth. Everyone should understand what they are putting in their mouths. Why? Educating yourself on nutrition basics and committing to implementing and enjoying this nutritious way of eating with mindfulness will enhance your life, extend your life, and may indeed save your life.

# WHY LEARN ABOUT NUTRITION?

The first way you can become a mindful eater is by learning some basics about nutrition. Now, before you indulge an urge to skip this section, we implore you to read ahead. Give yourself the chance to understand why some carbohydrates are health promoting and some are not, why some fats can be advantageous and nutritious while others are harmful, and why we generally eat too much protein and the potential dangers of doing so. The more you know about nutrition, the more likely you will be to eat healthy, and allow your body to run at its highest potential so you can live your best life. You will connect the way you feel—energetic instead of lethargic, buoyant instead of depressed—with the clean, wholesome foods you are eating.

Nutrition is a simple and sensible subject that need not be made overly complicated. The basic nutritional elements found in foods that contribute calories are protein, fat, and carbohydrates. In Phase Three of the Rice Diet, you will be eating a balance of 60 to 71 percent carbohydrate, 15 to 21 percent fat, and 14 to 18 percent protein for long-term weight loss and health maintenance. Fiber, a carbohydrate with no nutritional value per se, is also an important basic nutrition factor that we will discuss front and center. (Vitamins and minerals, and the health-promoting potential of antioxidants in particular, will be addressed in Chapter 8.)

# CARBOHYDRATES

Some of you may have been sucked into the carb paranoia and are wondering who is right, the pro-carb or anti-carb advocates. Quite simply, there is over a hundred years of clinical and epidemiological (population studies) research investigating the health advantages of a high-complex-carbohydrate diet versus the high-protein craze. The protein advocates have small clinical trials, showing that people do lose weight, but they lack scientific studies showing that people maintain their weight loss and health in the long-term. In contrast, the Rice Diet's six-year follow-up data show that a significant portion of our participants maintain their weights, or lose even more after leaving the program because they continue living the diet.

Like much in life, carbohydrates are not all good or all bad, but there are a lot of misconceptions about carbohydrates because of the fad diets that recommend extreme high-protein/high-fat and low-carbohydrate eating. The truth is that some kinds of carbohydrates promote health while others can trigger weight gain and the risk of chronic diseases such as diabetes and heart disease.

Our bodies prefer carbohydrates for energy, but it's the type of carbs we choose that is most important. Carbohydrates are classified into two main groups: simple carbohydrates (sugars) and complex carbohydrates (starches). Simple carbs are often described as "bad" and complex as "good." How do you know which is which? Does it ever really serve us to put things in such rigid boxes? Ask yourself the following:

• **Is it a sugar or a starch?** If the ingredient ends in "ose," it's a sugar.

• **Is it whole or is it processed?** If white, light, and fluffy, it's been processed into a simple carb containing a fraction of its natural nutrients and fiber.

• **How much fiber does it contain?** Fiber shields the starchy carbohydrates in food from immediate and rapid attack by digestive enzymes. This slows the release of sugar molecules into the bloodstream, gives you a sense of fullness, and aids in digestion.

Complex carbs are found in whole foods (i.e., any foods that are intact before cooking or eating them) including grains, beans, fruits, vegetables, and some nuts and seeds. Simple carbs are often found in processed food, which is defined as any food that has had its shape or form altered (grains versus flour, for example). Basically, the more whole or intact a food is, the better it is for you.

Another way to categorize and consider carbs is by their glycemic index and glycemic load. In short, the glycemic index (GI) measures the effect on blood glucose (or "blood sugar") of equivalent amounts of carbohydrates contained in different foods. The lower the GI of a food, the lower the blood glucose response, which is what you want. A GI of 55 or less is considered "low," meaning that it will cause less of a rise in blood glucose than a food with a high GI (>70).

Here are the factors that influence the GI of a food:

1. the type of fiber in the food, e.g., the higher the soluble fiber the lower the GI;

2. the form in which the food is eaten, e.g., rice cakes versus cooked brown rice or oatios versus steel-cut oats;

3. whether or not the food also contains fat;

4. the form of simple sugar present in the food, e.g. fructose versus glucose (with fructose causing less of an increase in blood glucose level);

5. the effect of protein and fat that are consumed along with the carbohydrate, and

6. the structure of starch that is contained in the carbohydrate of the food, e.g., foods with amylose (long, straight chains of glucose molecules) have a lower GI than foods with amylopectin (highly branched chains of glucose molecules).

So, given this, you can again see that high-fiber foods (whole fruits, vegetables, beans, and whole grains) will have a lower GI than highly processed low-fiber foods. But it's not just the quality of a food that influences your response to blood sugar. It's also the quantity of the carbohydrate in the foods you eat. In the late 1990s, researchers at Harvard University introduced the concept of glycemic load (GL) in an effort to quantify the overall glycemic effect of a portion of food.

A GL of 20 or more is considered high, 11 to 19 is medium, and a GL of 10 or less is low. Knowing the basic effect of a type of carbohydrate on blood glucose levels (GI) and factoring in a realistic portion size of a particular food (GL) are valuable in better predicting glycemic response. How does this affect you? Most of the participants dramatically improve their blood sugar levels, stabilize them, which reverses diabetic complications and helps with weight loss

Unfortunately, 85 percent of the grains and cereals consumed in the current U.S. diet are highly processed refined grains, which often have both high GI and GLs. Before the Industrial Revolution, all cereals were ground with stone milling tools, and unless the flour was sieved, it contained the entire contents of the grain: the germ, bran, and endosperm (the nutritive tissue in the seeds of most flowering plants). But with more mechanized inventions taking over by the late nineteenth century, the nutritional characteristics of milled grain changed dramatically because the germ and bran were removed in the milling process. So the next time you eat light, endosperm-only bread be mindful that you are among the first people in the history of the world to eat a fraction of a whole food. Ask yourself: Do you want to choose a grain product that now contains one-third of the nutrition it naturally offers?

The other result of an industrialized food supply is the seemingly insatiable appetite for refined sugar, also a carbohydrate. Increased sugar consumption in the last thirty years reflects a much larger worldwide trend that has occurred in Western nations since the Industrial Revolution, some 200 years ago. This is easy to believe when you observe how many people are consuming processed foods high in simple carbohydrates: sugar, high-fructose corn syrup, and white flour. The processing, a resulting reduction in fiber, causes these foods to have a higher glycemic index and often a higher glycemic

## MINDFULNESS TIP TO MEDITATE

The next time you are considering a simple sugar treat take a few deep breaths and ask yourself if you'd rather have that nutritionless sweet or the freshest, organic antioxidant-packed fruit you can get. Think about how your body feels when you eat fruit as opposed to refined sugar. Can you imagine the headaches, the cravings, and the anxiety sugar often produces? Let this awareness inspire the choice you truly desire.

load; they are absorbed quickly, inspiring spikes in blood glucose, which cause surges in insulin. These surges tend to cause a vicious cycle: subsequent sugar lows lead to increasing hunger and a strong desire to eat more simple carbohydrates. The resulting excessive insulin promotes atherosclerosis, the underlying cause of most heart disease, and increases the conversion of calories into triglycerides (fats in the blood). Over time insulin surges often lead to insulin resistance, causing further weight gain. Insulin may also raise our secretion of an enzyme (lipoprotein lipase), which increases the uptake of fat into cells, again leading to weight gain.

## GOOD CARBS TO EAT: THE MORE WHOLE THE BETTER

**Rich in Insoluble Fiber:**

Buckwheat groats

Bulgur (cracked wheat)

Quinoa

Amaranth

Millet

Couscous

Fregole

Rice

Whole grain bread (check the label to make sure that whole grain is the first ingredient)

**Rich in Soluble Fiber:**

Oat groats (whole oats), steel-cut oats, rolled, or oat bran

Polenta

Barley

Beans (legumes), lentils

Soybean products: Tempeh, edamame, or other whole soybean product

Most people realize their appetites are stimulated by sugar and refined flour. We have never seen a patient whose appetite was stimulated by fruits or complex carbohydrates (grains and cereals) while on the Rice Diet. Do we really need something to taste more deliciously sweet than fresh, cold watermelon, or the juice from one? When you're tempted, remind yourself to breathe and be conscious before you slurp down hundreds to thousands of calories in beverages or foods that are primarily refined sugar and chemicals. Breathe; be mindful about what you put in your body.

Our main advice is this: whenever possible, avoid highly processed grains, cereals, and sugars and instead eat minimally processed whole grains, fruits, and vegetables. A good general rule of thumb is to be sure that three-fourths or more of your grain intake is whole rather than processed and white and light.

# FIBER

You have probably heard a lot about the importance of fiber, but did you know that fiber is actually a form of a carbohydrate? Fiber is a carbohydrate that cannot be absorbed by humans. Like other carbohydrates, fiber contains 4 calories per gram, but those calories just pass right through you. That's why fiber is so good for your digestion—it helps move food through your system.

For decades the importance of fiber was overlooked because it can't be absorbed, and was thus considered an element of food with no redeeming nutritional value. In fact, during the industrial age, when we first learned how to remove fiber from our grains and cereals and make them white and light, eating processed food became a mark of sophistication. However, the outer husk, or bran, contains much of the grain's nutritional content, so this status symbol led to vitamin B deficiencies that caused nervous system damage, mental illness, and even death. Obviously, we learned to enrich processed grains with some nutrients that were stripped during the processing,

## MINDFULNESS TIP

You could eat no-fat, no-salt cream puffs plus a fiber pill or you could get much more nutritional boost from a *Blueberry-Banana Muffin,* page 289.

but even today these enriched grains are nutritionally inferior, and lacking greatly in the fiber department. The recommended daily intake of fiber is 38 grams per day for adult men and 25 grams per day for adult women, according to government nutrition experts. To put this into perspective, the average American (who typically has high cholesterol, out of control blood sugars, or some gut disorder) takes in only 14 grams per day. Vegetarians routinely consume 50 grams per day. However, the fiber intake of Paleolithic man, who had few of our chronic diseases, is estimated at 100 grams per day. So for people who are trying to eat healthier, we recommend an average of 30 to 50 grams or more of fiber per day.

# PROTEIN

Protein is an essential, important nutrient and probably the most overrated nutrient in our society. Although protein is necessary, too much can be harmful. There is a large amount of scientific evidence that links animal protein and accompanying saturated fat and cholesterol with heart disease and other chronic diseases. Excess protein may cause loss of calcium and decreased levels of urinary citrate, which can lead to osteoporosis and kidney stones. And remember, protein almost always comes with high amounts of saturated fat and sodium, as in meat and dairy. Even tofu, the vegetarian's delight, has more fat in it than hamburger. It is true that the fat in tofu is healthful compared to the fat in meat, but any fat still has 120 calories per tablespoon. Egg whites are a source of almost pure protein (the yolk is fat, mostly cholesterol). Fortunately, beans are high in not only protein, but in iron, calcium, potassium, and fiber with viscosity—thus, the perfect alternative to meat! Beans are a recommended daily component for all healthy diets.

Proteins are made of amino acids. Amino acids are simply the building blocks of protein. Human beings need twenty amino acids, and can make all but eight or nine of them from sugars and other amino acids. The eight to nine amino acids we can't make are called essential amino acids, and we have to eat them in plants or animals.

In order to eat complete proteins we need to complement grains that are typically low in one or more essential amino acids with another vegetarian food like beans that are high in them. Just remember that you need to eat whole grains and beans or dairy daily. The essential amino acids from yesterday's beans find today's amino acids from grains in an amino acid pool in your body. It's a no-brainer—who would want to eat beans without cornbread, corn chips, tortillas, nonfat yogurt (instead of sour cream) or rice anyway?

## QUINOA: A SUPER PROTEIN

Many people still believe that you have to be careful to get enough protein if you aren't eating animal products. This is far from the truth. All of the essential amino acids are found in the super grain quinoa. Considered a complete protein, it not only offers more than twice the protein and iron, but five times the magnesium and potassium of white rice. Quinoa is a grain truly worth trying. People like it because it has a very exotic mouth feel, or crunch to it. It is good with sweets, like *Quinoa Pudding* (page 293), or *Quinoa Veggie Salad* (page 223).

So please don't worry about whether or not you are getting sufficient protein on the Rice Diet. It has been shown that we only really need about 20 grams of protein per day. This 20 grams is enough to keep your body from using its own sources of protein (e.g., your muscles). Others have suggested that people losing weight need only 16 grams of protein per day to stay in nitrogen balance. The Basic Rice Diet supplies the necessary 16 grams of protein, practically all of it from the rice. And keep in mind that when readers eat the Lacto-Vegetarian Rice Diet for the other six days, they're averaging significantly more protein for the week, since vegetables and beans contain more protein than fruit.

Take the example of C., a twenty-year-old athlete who went on the Rice Diet and lost a total of 103 pounds in 161 days (0.64 pounds per day). His strength and endurance improved considerably. His ability to bench press increased from 285 to 370 pounds after losing the weight. As he explained, "In addition to all of this, my cardiovascular endurance has improved ten-fold. When I arrived, I could do no more than thirty minutes of any sort of cardio. Now, I am doing about four hours of cardio each day. Thanks for everything, Dr. Rosati." If this young man lost any muscle, it sure doesn't show up in his performance. Health-wise, his blood pressure went from 136/82 to 106/60 and his cholesterol fell from 183 to 129 while his good HDL-cholesterol went from 41 to 46. Clearly the amount of protein on the Rice Diet was sufficient! Again, on the Rice Diet, you get plenty of protein from grains, beans, and vegetables. If you really want to worry about protein, then worry about what comes along with the protein in your meat choices (i.e., excessive saturated fat, cholesterol, sodium, carcinogens, or maybe the risk of mad cow disease)!

When you graduate to Phase Three (maintenance), and if you feel you want more protein, add whole grains, beans, fish, nonfat dairy, other seafood, eggs (free-range, organic), poultry, or lean meats, preferably in that order, with respect to health. Again, if you want meat, make sure to stick with the leanest cuts: the round cut of beef, pork tenderloin, or, better yet, wild lean game. But if you are going to eat meat, first read *Fast Food Nation,* and keep an eye on your cholesterol!

Keep in mind, too, that there is no danger in a strict vegetarian diet if the person eats 800 calories or more, including plenty of beans and dark greens (if not beans, then an iron and calcium supplement), and whole grains. The only supplement he would need is the amount of vitamin $B_{12}$ in a multivitamin/mineral pill and an additional calcium supplement. Protein inadequacies are virtually impossible to experience unless you are literally starving to death (eating less than 500 calories per day), or consuming only foods without protein: fruit, fat, sugar, and alcohol. Yes, a Rum and Coke and Margarita Diet would do it!

## GOOD SOURCES OF PROTEIN

Dried beans and peas

Seafood, preferably fish

Eggs (organic, free-range are best; whites are lower in fat, cholesterol, and calories)

Wild game—such as venison (deer), buffalo, and boar. Most wild game is lean with the exception of duck.

Grains and vegetables to a lesser extent, especially quinoa

The following only if you think you can stop at 1 tablespoon:

Nuts and nut butters (beware: a tablespoon can lead many to eat in excess)

Seeds or butters such as tahini (sesame seed butter)

# SURPRISING SEAFOOD AND MEAT COMPARISONS

Serving size 3 ounces

| Seafood | Calories | Protein | Fat | Saturated Fat | Cholesterol | Sodium |
|---|---|---|---|---|---|---|
| Catfish | 120 | 19 | 5 | 1 | 60 | 65 |
| Clam, 12 sm. | 130 | 22 | 2 | 0 | 60 | 95 |
| Cod | 90 | 10 | 1 | 0 | 50 | 60 |
| Crab, blue | 90 | 19 | 1 | 0 | 80 | 310 |
| Crayfish | 96 | 20 | 1.2 | 0.3 | 149 | 57 |
| Flounder | 100 | 20 | 1 | 0 | 50 | 85 |
| Halibut | 120 | 22 | 2 | 0 | 30 | 60 |
| Haddock | 90 | 20 | 1 | 0 | 60 | 70 |
| Lobster | 100 | 20 | 1 | 0 | 100 | 320 |
| Mackerel | 190 | 21 | 12 | 3 | 60 | 95 |
| Mussel | 93 | 13 | 2.4 | 0.6 | 31 | 305 |
| Orange Roughy | 70 | 16 | 1 | 0 | 20 | 70 |
| Oyster, 12 med | 120 | 12 | 4 | 1 | 90 | 190 |
| Salmon, Atlantic Coho | 150 | 22 | 7 | 1 | 50 | 50 |

| | | | | | | |
|---|---|---|---|---|---|---|
| Sea Bass | 105 | 20 | .6 | 2.2 | 45 | 4 |
| Scallop (6 lg. or 14 sm.) | 150 | 29 | 1 | 0 | 60 | 275 |
| Shrimp | 115 | 23 | 2 | 0.4 | 164 | 159 |
| Tuna (yellowfin) | 118 | 25 | 1 | 0 | 48 | 39 |
| Tuna, light, chunk Starkist | 90 | 20 | 1.5 | 0.3 | 30 | 465 |
| Tuna, white, chunk Starkist | 105 | 23 | 1.5 | 0.3 | 30 | 45 |
| Crown Prince Albacore Tuna, no salt added, ¼ cup | 60 | 14 | 0 | 0 | 20 | 30 |
| Crown Prince Alaskan Pink Salmon, wild, ¼ cup | 80 | 10 | 4.5 | 1 | 15 | 50 |
| Crown Prince Kipper Snacks, naturally smoked, 1 can, 3.25 oz | 190 | 19 | 13 | 2 | 60 | 70 |
| Haddon House Fillets of Mackerel, water packed, ¼ cup | 90 | 14 | 4.5 | 1.5 | 35 | 55 |
| Season Sardines, no salt added, 1 can, 4.25 oz. | 130 | 22 | 5 | 3 | 35 | 50 |
| Chicken, light | 186 | 34 | 5 | 1.3 | 90 | 76 |
| Turkey, light | 184 | 35 | 6 | 1.9 | 89 | 82 |
| Pork tenderloin | 194 | 34 | 5.7 | 2 | 110 | 79 |
| Beef, round | 164 | 27 | 5.3 | 2 | 72 | 53 |

Jean A.T. Pennington. *Journal of the American Dietetic Association* (October 1992): 1254; and data from food labels.

# FAT, FAT, AND MORE FAT

Fat comes in different shapes and sizes but all fatty acids fall into one of two basic categories: saturated or unsaturated. Saturated, monounsaturated, and polyunsaturated fatty acids are the building blocks of all fats.

• **Saturated fatty acids** are by far highest in animal products, with the exception of seafood, which is low in saturated fats. Although some saturated fatty acids are more dangerous than others, high-saturated fat intake is still the most clear predictor of who will have high cholesterol and heart disease.

• **Monounsaturated fats** are undoubtedly the most healthful. Olive oil, then canola (rapeseed oil) are our first and second recommendations for you; olive oil is the highest in monounsaturated fats and canola the lowest in saturated fats.

• **Polyunsaturated fats** are a mixed bag. This category contains the incredibly beneficial omega-3 fatty acid–rich fish oils (known as EPA and DHA), and the excessively consumed omega-6 fatty acid–rich foods, such as oils from corn, safflower, soybean, sunflower, and cottonseed. The latter you may recognize from the many processed food labels, which are usually preceded by the words "partially hydrogenated." Hydrogenation of an oil creates what is called a "trans fat," which is thought to be potentially even more harmful than the naturally occurring saturated-fat foods. Food scientists call hydrogenated fats "plasticized fats"—need I say more?!

• **Essential fatty acids,** or EFAs, are polyunsaturated fatty acids that are necessary for normal growth and development; our bodies cannot manufacture them, which means we must get them from our diet. There are two families of EFAs, omega-6 fatty acids and omega-3 fatty acids. Most of us are getting far more omega-6 fatty acids than we need. Omega-6 fatty acids are most abundant in common vegetable oils: corn, safflower, sunflower, and cottonseed oils. They are also found in high amounts in grain-fed animal meat, which constitutes most of the meat eaten in the United States.

The omega-6 fatty acid–rich oils are commonly used in processed foods because the oils are cheaper. Since processed foods have become such a large proportion of the average industrial nation's intake, the omega-3 fatty acid intake has gone down and the omega-6 fatty acid intake has increased. Research suggests that if you want to enhance your chances for optimal health, you should have a diet with a ratio of omega-6 to omega-3 fatty acids that is less than four to one. However, the average American's diet contains from fourteen to twenty times more omega-6 than omega-3 fatty acids, which greatly increases the chronic diseases of our civilization. In the 1970s, numerous studies started pointing to the correlation between omega-6 fatty acids and an increase in cancer. The first large study to show a link was in a Los Angeles veterans' hospital in the 1970s, where a group of men assigned to a diet high in omega-6 oils experienced twice the number of cancer deaths as those on a more traditional diet. But despite this and the many other studies suggesting this correlation, the majority still feast on convenience foods loaded with these omega-6 fatty acid–rich oils.

By far, the majority of omega-3 fats are found in seafood (especially fatty fish), with lesser amounts found in green leafy vegetables (especially purslane, which cannot be easily bought in the U.S. yet, but if you can find the seeds it's easy to grow), flaxseed (freshly ground), walnuts, and canola (rapeseed oil). Omega-3 fatty acids are a type of polyunsaturated fat thought to be beneficial for preventing heart disease and numerous risk factors. Some studies show omega-3 fatty acids lower cholesterol, but most of them show more significant reductions in blood pressure and triglycerides. Omega-3 fatty acids also help prevent blood clots and coronary artery spasms, which are two underlying causes of heart attacks. High amounts of omega-3 fatty acids are found in oilier fish such as mackerel, salmon, trout, bluefish, and tuna. No one really knows whether the inclusion of seafood is better or worse for your heart than a strict vegetarian diet, but seafood is indisputably the best meat choice.

# COMPARISON OF DIETARY FAT

Not all fat is alike. The amount of saturated fat you eat is the best predictor of an increase in cholesterol, and thus, risk of heart disease. All fats have a combination of saturated, polyunsaturated, and monounsaturated fatty acids, but you want the least amount of saturated fat as possible. Although there are fatty acids within each group

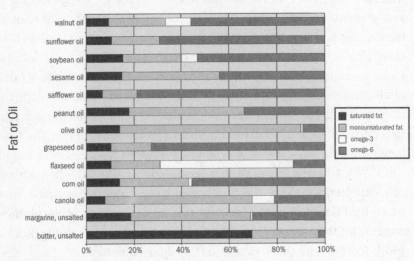

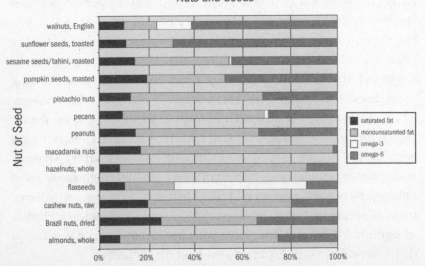

that are more or less health promoting, in general, it is to your advantage to choose the foods (oils, nuts and seeds, meats, and seafoods) with the lowest percentage of saturated fat and omega-6 fatty acids and the highest percentage of monounsaturated and omega-3 fatty acids.

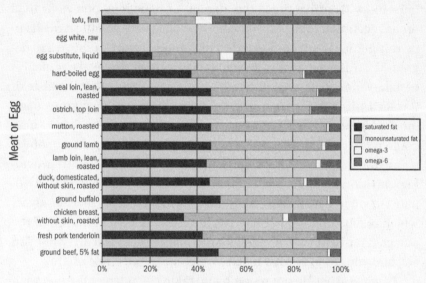

Meats and Eggs

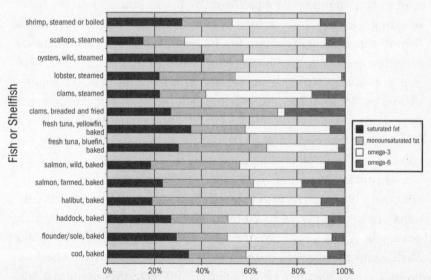

Fish and Shellfish

Charts derived from U.S.D.A. data.

Dr. Artemis Simopoulos, in her book *The Omega Diet* (Harper-Perennial, 1999), advises people to eat fish three to five times per week. If you don't care for fish, you will benefit by daily increasing your intake of flaxseed oil, ground flaxseeds, canola oil, walnut oil or walnuts, or you can supplement with fish oils. Flaxseed oil contains more than five times the amount of beneficial omega-3s than other vegetarian foods do, but since the oil is very volatile it needs to be refrigerated, and not heated to high temperatures (above 210 degrees F.). Adding a freshly ground tablespoon of flaxseed per meal is certainly more palatable for most people who report that the taste of flaxseed oil is too strong and fishy smelling. Another more commonly consumed product that has a significant omega-3 fatty acid content are the Gold Circle Farm eggs. This company, and hopefully a growing number of other chicken farms, are dedicated to providing nutritionally enhanced eggs from chickens that are fed an all-natural, plant-based diet. They feed their chickens marine algae, which results in eggs that have eight times the concentration of the omega-3 fat DHA than a regular supermarket egg. You are what you eat, and your food is what it eats. Welcome to the circle of life!

In general, we do not recommend taking supplements other than a multivitamin mineral supplement. We prefer you get into the habit of eating omega-3s in your food sources, but you may prefer taking a fish oil supplement. They are available at all groceries and pharmacies; the tip on page 89 for assessing their cost may be helpful. There is a potentially bewildering variety of names for fish oil supplements, but look for the contents to read the two particular omega-3 fatty acids: the EPA and DHA we have abbreviated for simplicity's sake should be confirmed on the bottle; they stand for "eicosapentaenoic acid" and "docosahexaenoic acid."

As previously stated, your body functions best when your diet contains a balanced ratio of fatty acids. The typical Western diet contains approximately 14 to 20 times more omega-6 fatty acids than omega-3s. A few years ago, the Lyon Diet Heart Study found that a Mediterranean olive oil–based diet, with an omega-6 to omega-3 ratio of 4:1, had phenomenally beneficial effects. Although the Mediterranean diet contained 35 percent fat, it contained less meat, and more fish, grains, fruits, and vegetables than the typical American diet.

The Lyon Diet Heart Study made medical history. Those on the olive oil–based diet had an unprecedented 76 percent lower risk of dying from cardiovascular disease or suffering heart failure, heart attack, or stroke! The news was sensational: an age-old diet had proven more effective at saving lives than any other heart diet, drug, lifestyle program, or any combination of these elements. In addition to the above improvements, their studies also showed that the diet made you less vulnerable to inflammatory and autoimmune diseases. You may even be less prone to mental disorders such as depression and Alzheimer's disease with the Mediterranean approach.

To reduce weight and chronic diseases, you can choose between very low-fat (Asian-like) diets, or much higher, healthier fat-rich Mediterranean diets. It's really what you think you will be more likely to do for the duration; you may choose to do a combination of the two.

## OMEGA-3 FATTY ACID SUPPLEMENT COST ANALYSIS

To assess the costs of your omega-3 supplements, use the following formula: add up the amount of EPA and DHA per capsule, then multiply by the number of capsules in the bottle, and then divide by the cost. This gives you the cost per milligram. To convert this to the cost per gram, which is the recommended daily dose, multiply by 1,000 (move the decimal point three spaces to the right).

# Fats—How Low Should You Go?

The answer to this question depends upon who you ask. We believe that how much a person should limit fat intake is dependent on disease risk factors, weight loss goals, and what that person will commit to. Given how strongly high-fat diets correlate to increased risk for obesity and the diseases correlated with it, including certain types of cancer, and heart disease, the lower the fat the better for those in these groups. The research has actually shown that arteries can widen and heart disease can be reversed by eating less than 20 percent fat diets. Dr. Dean Ornish's study showed such benefits in the majority of those who ate less than 10 percent fat diets, as Ricers do on Phases One and Two, while Dr. Schuler's study showed improvements in subjects eating a diet with less than 20 percent fat, more like our maintenance Phase Three. So the more risk factors of heart disease you have, the more reasons you have to eat less fat. Readers who want to keep their fat intake to 10 to 20 percent can refer to my previous book, *Heal Your Heart* (Wiley, 1997). In addition, inexpensive calorie, fat, and sodium counting books can be purchased at most drug stores, pharmacies, or bookstores.

# No Dangers of "Too Low Fat" on a Whole Foods Diet

The average person does not need to consume more than 14 grams of fat per day to meet the daily requirements of essential fatty acids. This amount of fat can be found naturally in seven ½-cup servings of starchy foods, without adding any oil. It is almost impossible to get an essential fatty acid deficiency in someone with a functioning mouth and gut.

Since fat (whether saturated, monounsaturated, or polyunsaturated) has nine calories per gram, over twice the amount of calories

# INSPIRATIONAL CORNER

D.J. was twenty-five when he came to see us in May 1990. He had symptoms of sleep apnea (falling asleep during the day). His weight was 492, his blood pressure 156/94, and his cholesterol 240. After four weeks, he had lost 59 pounds. By August 31, his weight was 355. He had lost 137 pounds in 105 days. His cholesterol was down to 183.

By December 11, his weight was 275. He had lost 217 pounds in less than seven months. At one point, he got down to about 190 but got into bodybuilding and as of July 2002, he was 260 pounds of muscle with a 34-inch waist.

S.Q. was sent here by his brother to prepare for a hip replacement. He walked with a cane. He had high blood pressure (168/100 on medications) and an enlarged heart (18.4 centimeter). His exercise was swimming. He lost 145 pounds in 245 days. His blood pressure was 94/60 without medications. He no longer needed his cane and did not need hip surgery until five years later (he had gained 10 pounds in this interval).

found in protein and carbohydrates, limiting fat is the obvious way to limit our calories. And research in the real world shows that people who have maintained significant weight losses for long periods of time eat a low-fat diet. In 1993, Dr. James Hill of the University of Colorado and Dr. Rena Wing of the University of Pittsburgh founded the National Weight Control Registry, a national database of people successful at maintaining a significant weight loss. Subjects have lost 30 pounds and kept it off for one year or longer, are eighteen years of age or older, and have completed lifestyle questionnaires initially and annually. The majority continue to report that low-fat diets are the key for successful weight loss and maintenance.

Fad diet books that demonize a particular macronutrient have really done a disservice to everyone who wants to lose weight, because they obscure the true root cause of obesity and resulting chronic diseases. The Rice Diet Program works long-term. Considering the fact that lifelong Ricers vary greatly in the percentage of calories they get from protein, fat, and carbohydrate, it's obvious to us

## A REVIEW OF YOUR RICE DIET DIETARY GUIDELINES

1. Be mindful of the foods you are eating.

2. Minimize fat intake, and make monounsaturated oil, such as olive oil and canola oil, your primary fats.

3. Eat foods rich in omega-3 fatty acids, such as fatty fish (mackerel, salmon, tuna, trout, and herring), walnuts, flaxseeds, green leafy vegetables, and eggs (free-range, organic). Take omega-3 supplements only if you cannot consistently enjoy fish three to five times per week.

4. Eat seven or more fresh servings of fruits and vegetables each day, organic whenever possible, preferably ones that are dark orange, red, or green.

5. Limit saturated fat (high in meats and dairy), and trans or partially hydrogenated fats (found in just about everything processed), and omega-6 fatty acids (high in corn, safflower, sunflower, soybean, and cottonseed oils) whenever possible.

6. Enjoy more vegetable proteins rich in fiber with beneficial viscosity (any dried bean or pea, oat or barley product).

that the key to weight loss and resulting health is the serious reduction of sodium, saturated fats, and refined (or processed) carbohydrates.

# Choosing to be a Conscious Consumer

We strongly believe that children are never too young to be taught about their food choices and the truth about the consequences of their choices in promoting health or disease when consumed regularly. As most educators and parents realize, it is far easier to learn desirable eating behaviors and habits initially rather than to relearn or change habits that are not health promoting later. If the adult shares the nutrition information in an empowering, fun way, most children will be open to exploring healthy new foods.

When our six-year-old begged me to buy him Gummy Bears, I (Kitty) chose not to totally restrict his freedom to select his dietary delights for himself. When we got home, I gave him six or seven Gummy Bears on a plate and he ate them with much satisfaction. The next day I came in and his dad had given him about six times as many! Knowing that he would not benefit by hearing my judgment of his dad's serving size selection, I later asked his dad to get conscious of how many Gummy Bears he had heaped on our son's plate, when he had been just as happy, if not happier, with one-sixth the amount the day before. Well, the next day I returned home to what at first seemed a repeat, his dad had supersized him another plate of Gummy Bears. I resisted the temptation to remove the Gummy Bears; I realized I needed to educate and empower my child to make his own conscious food choices.

I asked Chess if he knew what he was eating and how they made Gummy Bears. He, of course, said he did not. I proceeded to share how food labels are required to give us a list of the ingredients that are found in the food, and listed in the order they come by weight. His inquiring mind immediately wanted to know.

"Mmmm, let's see: sugar, which originally came from sugar cane . . . it offers calories, but no nutritional value. It's not great in excess, but it's not the worst thing in the world either; high-fructose corn syrup, again, is an empty calorie food that is thought to contribute to obesity and trick our body into thinking it is full when it has not really had any nutrition; gelatin . . . Chess, do you know what this is? . . . It's made from ground cow hooves and horns."

Chess looked at me with the most incredulous expression I had seen from him and asked if I was kidding. I calmly said no, that that was what they made it from. Then, I simply continued to define, in an age-appropriate fashion, what he was eating. The next day, Bob again gave Chess twenty-six Gummy Bears. Chess returned twenty-two. "Thanks, Daddy. I'm limiting myself to four per day now." Now, at age nine, he rarely asks for Gummy Bears!

In addition to the nutrition information previously described, today's mindful eater will also benefit from exploring information on where our food comes from, how it is grown and harvested or prepared, how it is preserved (or not), and how it gets to us.

In 2001 the United States Department of Agriculture (USDA) established a national standard to define organically produced foods. The complete USDA definition is more than 500 pages long, but basically it states that organic food must be produced without irradiation, the use of sewage sludge, genetically modified organisms (GMO), most conventional pesticides, and the aid of synthetic fertilizers. Organic meat and poultry are not to be given antibiotics and hormones or fed anything that is not 100 percent organic feed. Although you may have heard that organic labeling does not really guarantee that it is organic, the guidelines do offer us significant protection. While the guidelines are less than ideal, we are all responsible to be vocal with our politicians who create such loopholes, or fail to.

We choose to buy organic whenever we can. If you are fortunate enough to live near organic farms, you can visit and find out firsthand about what you are eating. Recently, we surfed the Internet and discovered that a nearby organic farm will deliver fresh vegetables right to our door every week. Now we all look forward to Thursdays!

Find out about the differences between these types of food and those we traditionally consume. Greg Hottinger's book *The Best Natural Foods on the Market Today* includes a nice practical summary on this topic. It helps you prioritize what foods are most important to buy organic. You have the most to gain by buying organic meats, milk, eggs, yogurt, cheese, and other dairy products. And the Environmental Working Group estimates that you can lower your pesticide exposure by 90 percent if you replace the top-twelve most contaminated fruits and vegetables with the least contaminated. The most pesticide-contaminated fruits and vegetables, if you don't buy organic, are peaches, strawberries, apples, spinach, nectarines, celery, pears, cherries, potatoes, sweet bell peppers, raspberries, and grapes. Some of the least pesticide-contaminated fruits and vegetables, if you don't buy organic, are pineapple, cauliflower, mango, sweet peas, asparagus, onions, broccoli, bananas, kiwi, tangerines, cabbages, and blueberries. Washing all nonorganic fruits and vegetables with soap and water is also important to remember.

We used to think we didn't have to be concerned about mercury in fish if we just ate farm-raised fish. Then, we became aware that farm-raised fish might be treated with chemicals and be raised without being able to swim. So now, we pretty much eat wild fish lower on the food chain, and eat sparingly of larger fatty fish such as swordfish and tuna. The bottom line is to choose to be conscious of what goes in your mouth. You are fully responsible for the food you choose to eat, and how this affects plants, animals, your community, and the planet.

Consider this: If you are drinking cow's milk that is not organic, it most likely came from cows that have been bred to produce greater and greater amounts of milk, with today's average cow producing six to eight gallons of milk each day, compared to only one and one-half gallons 100 years ago. And do you know about the highly controversial bovine somatotropin (BST, also called bovine growth hormone, BGH) injections that can increase milk yield by nearly a gallon per day? This is being injected into cows without labeling guidelines that would require producers to indicate the presence of BGH. Again, it's in your best interest to buy organic milk from companies like Organic Valley Farmers!

For far more sobering and graphic examples to inspire healthy eating choices, please read or watch the video of *Diet for a New America* by John Robbins. Another inspiring educational venue to explore is the Slow Food movement; check the Internet for your local chapter's events. It is much easier to appreciate a delicious organic apple after experiencing a local apple tasting with a grower whose life passion is to grow the greatest variety of organic apples in your state. Educating yourself on the healthiest foods available in your area can be an absolute joy! Yummy foods and a conscious community!

Regardless of your religion or philosophy, whether you call it "being responsible for your actions" or karma reward or debt, we are all connected and responsible for what we choose to consume and the consequences of these choices. Again, the more you know about what you eat, the better your choices will be.

As you continue your journey with us, remember that the Rice Diet is a lifestyle choice that inspires and challenges you to practice a mindfully consumed whole food plan that will fuel your body, mind, and spirit to their full potential.

# CHAPTER FIVE

# MAKE TIME FOR YOURSELF AND CREATE THE LIFE YOU WANT

*The solution to the problem of the day is the awakening of the consciousness of humanity to the divinity within.*

—HAZRAT INAYAT KHAN

Congratulations! You are moving right along in your journey to becoming truly mindful and fully yourself. You have begun the Rice Diet, changing the way you eat, and have begun losing weight. No doubt you feel better—perhaps leaner, stronger, and more energetic. Indeed, by becoming a mindful eater, informed about food, you are closer to deciding what you want to do with your weight, health, and life dreams.

Most diets begin and end at this point: they give you directions, descriptions of foods to eat, and then some encouragement to "just do it." And that is why we believe most diets fail.

At the Rice Diet Program, we believe strongly that in order to make this diet—or any diet for that matter—really livable, you need to become not only mindful of the food you put into your mouth but mindful of yourself and your life. It is when this mindfulness occurs that people begin not only to choose to eat differently but to live differently. This is where the sticking power of the diet takes root in your *dieta*, or way of living. In the last chapter, you took your first step of mindfulness by educating yourself about nutrition. By becoming more conscious and aware of the foods that you are eating and how they affect your body, you maximize your commitment to your new way of healthy eating, which will lead to weight loss. Now it's time to take a step further toward mindfulness by prioritizing "alone" time so you can rest, reflect, and renew.

The power of rest—and its benefits—cannot be underestimated. In our fast-paced, overscheduled society, it is rare that people actually take the time to rest at all, never mind on a daily basis. Yet we know that in order to stay healthy, the body needs its sleep. But rest is more than sleep; rest is ridding your body of stress, letting it relax, reflect, and renew. Exercise can inspire this renewal for you. Mind-body activities such as yoga and meditation can also assist you in achieving this regenerative need. And simply taking time to think can do this for you. We used to say six days of exercise a week were enough; even God rested on the seventh day. But why should we take a day off from taking care of ourselves?

When the body is able to relax, the mind does so, too. And when your body and mind are able to reach this state of restfulness, all sorts of wonderful things can happen:

• **Your body becomes healthier and you feel physically stronger and more supple.**

• **You feel more connected to your body's signals of hunger and fullness.**

• **Your rate of weight loss continues to increase because your body feels safe to release it.**

• **You feel less stressed, so you will be less likely to turn to food as a stress-response.**

• **Thoughts and feelings are more easily managed, allowing you to respond calmly rather than react impulsively to stressors.**

• **Your mind stays more clear and less anxious, enabling you to stay focused on your commitment to your diet.**

First focus on figuring out a way to rest that works for you, and second, become aware of your self once you reach this state of internal peace. Each of us has the power to create time for ourselves, whether that is spent exercising, meditating, doing yoga or tai chi, or simply being quiet with yourself. When you make this time for yourself, a miraculous, life-changing thing begins to occur: you hear the true voice within you. Are you ready to listen?

# MEDITATION AND CONSCIOUS BREATHING

Meditation simply means quiet time in which you calm your body and clear your mind. People meditate for long periods of time or just for moments squeezed into the day while sitting in traffic, waiting in line at the grocery store, or by taking a moment to be still at our desk. Meditation can occur during prayer, a walk in the woods, or the simple act of watching the leaves fall or the fire flicker or the ocean waves ascend and descend.

The actual technique of meditation begins with becoming aware of your breath. This can be as simple as "Breathe in: 'I know that I am breathing in.' Breathe out: 'I know that I am breathing out.' " By focusing on your breath (the technique of conscious breathing), you naturally quiet the mind so you can see yourself and the world around you more clearly. With this calmness and clarity, you are then able to look deeply into yourself, becoming aware of your thoughts, feelings, bodily sensations, and anything that interests you or warrants your attention. Once you look deeply, you are able to achieve better understanding, and it is this understanding that leads to transformation. The more comfortable you become with this process, the less attached you become to the content of your thoughts, and through this nonattachment, peace ensues—peace of mind and peace of body.

There are many benefits from meditation. While calming the mind, it allows us to reconnect with our bodies. One of the main reasons that we do not take better care of our bodies is that we live in our minds. The breath ties the mind and the body back together. As we become more aware of our body, we take better care of it. In the

West, meditation has been popularized as a stress management technique, which it definitely is, and one way to connect to your body through your mind is through an exercise called the body scan. In *Full Catastrophe Living*, Jon Kabat-Zinn describes such a technique in the stress management course that he has developed, as well as in his CDs. This course has been replicated in many settings and may be available in your area. Sister Jina demonstrates a body scan exercise on the CD *Plum Village Meditations with Thich Nhat Hanh* (see Appendix B). In this body scan, you are instructed to breathe in, bringing awareness to your body or a part of your body; when you exhale, you smile, thanking that part of your body. Through this exercise, you come to appreciate that each and every part of you is a miracle. We also recommend tapes or CDs by Jon Kabat-Zinn (see Appendix B) to help you with the body scan and meditation. At the very least, these exercises are quite relaxing.

But for anyone on the quest to lose weight, the ultimate goal of meditation is that it can lead you to make a conscious change in your behavior; this is the end result of transformation. One story Thich Nhat Hanh tells on the CD *Truly Seeing* sums up the experience of each mindful participant in the Rice Diet Program. He tells the story of a river, born as a stream, that sings and dances down the mountain wanting to get quickly to the ocean. Though she looks happy, she is unaware that she is happy and so is not really happy. The river is emblematic of the dieter who loses weight quickly, but doesn't enjoy it because she is only interested in getting to her goal. Then, the river gets to the lowlands and slows down, thinking it will take forever to get to the ocean. In the same way, as the dieter's weight loss slows, she starts thinking it will take forever to get to her goal. It is at this point that the river (and the dieter) begin to suffer. The river gets distracted when she sees the clouds. She chases them, but they are fickle and never stay for long. When they disappear from her view, her suffering returns. The dieter, meanwhile, is chasing the thin person who appears in her mind, but then vanishes, leaving her disenchanted and frustrated.

Then a strong wind comes and blows away all the clouds, leaving the river alone with her miserable thoughts. But, that night, with no clouds to distract her, the river is alone to focus on herself: in the stillness she realizes that she *is* water, the same as clouds and the ocean. And with that she sees that what she has been chasing has always been within her.

The next morning, the river awakes to see the beautiful blue sky that she has never noticed before. She is suddenly able to enjoy the present moment.

And the dieter? When things slow down in her mind and she returns to herself, she realizes that the thin person she is seeking is already there within her. Suddenly, she begins to enjoy the present moment, breathing, exercising, and taking nourishing food. When she is present, her transformation takes place. For the dieter, meditation, or simply being quiet in her mind—to see her thoughts, feelings, and self with nonattachment—lets the person within her come to her.

Meditation leads to mindfulness. You become present and the object of your awareness becomes present. When you are present and your mind is calm, you see clearly. When you see clearly, you are less attached to your self, your thoughts, your feelings so that you can then see and experience yourself more clearly. This clarity, in turn, enables you to look deeply into yourself, understand yourself, and make decisions to change behaviors that are no longer working for you. This is how—and where—true healing takes place.

We have witnessed again and again the benefits of meditation our participants at the Rice Diet Program have experienced, and know that you can reach this state of peace, calm, and knowingness, too. Ricers still find they have a lot of time on their hands when they're not spending so much time eating. They use it to rest, relax, and become mindful in order to have losing weight be a conscious choice as well as an activity. They have a lot of opportunity to notice when their thoughts turn to food, and sense how they truly are feeling and responding to life. They might say to themselves, "Well, if I'm not really hungry, then what am I feeling?" Meditation allows your real thoughts and feelings to surface. Once this is allowed, or is given

## MEDITATION EXERCISES AND CDS

Thich Nhat Hanh's *Blooming of a Lotus* offers many meditations to calm the mind and body, to look deeply, and to heal. Indeed, we cannot recommend enough Thich Nhat Hanh's books, audio books, and talks to help you apply meditation and mindfulness to your personal journey.

time to happen, your relationship with food is more clear: you eat when you're hungry and stop when you're full.

The key is not to overthink the idea of meditation. Meditation is simply the process of quieting the mind. When the mind is quiet, you feel peaceful. End of story. But by doing meditation in whichever way is calming, for as little or as long as you want, you will begin to hear yourself and know yourself. And that's when your transformation begins to take root, to anchor, to create a firm foundation upon which to weather life's storms.

# WHAT IS YOGA?

Yoga is an ancient form of meditation in motion. For thousands of years, people have been practicing the yoga asanas (poses) and other meditative principles of yoga to clear their minds, strengthen and tone their bodies, and achieve balance in their lives. The goal of yoga is to reach balance of the mind and body. It is also a more comfortable, logical entry into meditation for those more accustomed to *doing* than *being*.

Here at the Rice Diet Program, our esteemed colleague, Joy Anandi, has developed Flowing Gentle Path Yoga, a yoga that is suitable for people who have never done yoga or who are limited in their ability to move because of their overweight state. Flowing Gentle Path Yoga is a system of yoga therapy that involves a whole body workout (even sitting in a large armless chair or wheelchair), using the ancient system of Pranayama (breath control) and Hatha Yoga (physical exercise).

Joy created this system at the Rice Diet Program beginning in 1993. Her system of flowing with the breath releases tension on the cellular level. When the breath and the movement are of the same duration, the exercise becomes meditation in motion. Breathing is the key to quieting the mind, so always be aware of your breath and its quality.

The practice of yoga includes gentle stretches, breathing, relaxation, visualization, and meditation. Participants are encouraged to either use a floor mat or a chair; both ways are acceptable. Through these techniques, you can make more conscious choices to respond rather than to react to stress, and bring the nervous system back into balance.

The physical stretches of yoga asanas bring you back in touch with your physical body where people tend to register and retain stress and emotion. The movements are done deliberately and meditatively. In various positions, the spine is massaged by bending forward, back, laterally, and through gentle twisting. These stretches are never done to the point of strain. Through these movements, you are able to develop a strong, limber body with fewer chronic aches and pains, to stimulate and improve the glandular system, to release tensions held in your muscles, and to bring a sense of ease and relaxation back into your body.

You do not have to be an expert to enjoy the wondrous benefits of yoga. As soon as you begin doing a simple, gentle practice you will begin to feel better. It is not recommended to eat before you meditate or practice yoga. You should wait at least two to three hours after a heavy meal or one and a half hours after a light meal.

Yoga is a technique ideally suited to prevent physical and mental illness and to protect the body, generally, developing an inevitable sense of self-reliance and assurance. By its very nature, it is inextricably associated with universal laws: respect for life, truth, and patience are all indispensable factors in the drawing of a quiet breath, in calmness of mind, and firmness of will.

—*Yehudi Menuhin*, Why Yoga?

Yoga is a means of getting back in touch with yourself. Its practice can help you to quiet yourself, ease your body and your mind, and let you access your inherent peace and power by encouraging you to stay present. You will immediately begin to get a better understanding of how every thought and emotion you experience affects every cell of your body. It's true—yoga can create health! Since yoga is based on this interconnectedness of the body, breath, emotions, thoughts, and immune system, each of these elements is touched by yoga. This makes yoga a valuable aid in stress management, complementing Western approaches to medical care. It helps you to relax in any situation, to be less controlled by your habits, and to be more at peace with life.

The practice of meditation or yoga does not require a belief in religion, or interfere with any religious practice. Meditation and yoga can assist you in acquiring a stable mind and a healthy body, so that you can achieve what is important to you and live life in a more meaningful way. Many people, however, have found that both have helped them deepen their own religious practices and prayer.

Yoga can assist in weight loss through its stimulation of the endocrine system and its effect on metabolism. It is a great weight-bearing and muscle and bone strengthening exercise, thus helpful in preventing osteoporosis. It's also easy to do anywhere and requires no special equipment. All you need is a quiet place, loose fitting, comfortable clothes, and a cushioned area on the floor large enough for you to spread out, or a comfortable chair.

No longer is yoga just for people who have visited India, the birthplace of yoga. Thankfully, yoga studios and classes are popping up all over the United States. Check one out near you and join the flow! If you cannot find a class in your community, many yoga experts offer CDs and DVDs that you can follow in the comfort of your own home. (See Appendix B.)

## INSPIRATIONAL CORNER

When L.B. came to the Rice Diet Program, she was a desperate woman, having gained over 200 pounds and recently taken a serious fall. Her diabetes and blood pressure were out of control. She came in on a walker and could not drive. Her doctor suggested, then lovingly insisted, that she come to the program. She agreed to come for one month. She attended all the classes and stayed faithful to the program.

By the end of the month, she felt so much better she wanted to stay longer. With the blessings of her husband and family, she decided to stay as long as it took to get the job done. She attended the yoga classes and says they've played a major role in her recovery.

L.B. now demonstrates yoga poses for other people in chairs. She has more flexibility than she ever thought possible and can stand on her feet for the standing poses. To date she has lost 143 pounds, is off all blood pressure and diabetes medications. As she says, "I feel as well as I did when I was twenty years old. What can I say? I have my life back! *Thank you Rice Diet Program and thank you, Joy Anandi, for giving me back my life!*"

# TAI CHI

Another way Ricers make time to rest and restore themselves is through the ancient Chinese movement art, T'ai-chi Ch'üan, which dates back over three thousand years. Dr. Jay Dunbar teaches an inspired class that is based on the Chinese view of the body as an energy system. T'ai-chi Ch'üan brings together many aspects of Chinese culture: medicine, martial arts, Taoist philosophy, meditation, and calisthenics. Though the Rice Diet Program is firmly rooted in Western medicine, we offer tai chi because other views of self and healing are both possible and useful in your weight loss process.

When most people think of tai chi they think of groups of people moving in slow synchronization in the parks, but tai chi also includes seated and standing meditation, a wide range of auxiliary exercises (including stretching, joint warm-ups, massage, breathing, torso work), and movements based on the imitation of animals. The seated, standing, and moving exercises of tai chi can entertain, challenge, and fascinate—at all levels of human experience—physically, emotionally, and spiritually.

Experienced teachers of tai chi, such as our Dr. Jay, articulate an alternative perspective and make it inspiring. A typical class begins with a series of joint warm-ups, working from toes to ankles, through a knee massage and gentle undulations of the spine all the way up the torso, out the arms, and down to the fingers. Most classes include an introduction to some aspect of Chinese language, medical theory, personal energetics, or tai chi. The rest of the class is spent doing some kind of gentle, continuous movement, using simple qigong (energy work) or the opening movements of a tai chi form.

Though tai chi may sound foreign to you, consider this: The Rice Diet Program population is generally composed of highly intelligent people who are dealing with various life-threatening conditions, or conditions that they realize have adversely begun to affect their health or quality of life. Many have not engaged in any exercise for a long time, have a fear of failure, a lack of confidence in their ability to participate in more vigorous exercise programs, or a genuine inability to stand, to balance, or to move for any length of time. However, nearly all of those who have attended Dr. Jay's hour-plus weekly tai chi sessions have one thing in common: a sincere appreciation that they have been open enough to explore a practice that has assisted them in their quest for balance, centeredness, renewed wellness, and a revitalized lifestyle.

# GET MOVING

Beyond yoga and tai chi, traditional exercise is another way you can make time for yourself each day and increase your weight loss. You may not think of exercise as either restful or relaxing. And yet it inspires both. As your body becomes more conditioned, it is able to relax, replenishing your energy—both physical and mental. Of course, more traditional forms of exercise have other added benefits: they burn calories, improve your overall physical condition and immunity, and increase your ability to lose weight. As one participant pointed out, "I have tried many other diets before and they never worked. I always put the weight back on. The Rice Diet Program addresses the other components that make the diet possible for me in the long-term. I have never taken to meditation or yoga, but I now exercise regularly. I walk, lift weights, and even play tennis. I also know how to manage my stress. That has made all the difference." So for those of you who are not yet interested in trying meditation, yoga, or tai chi, traditional exercise (walking, swimming, or other sports) is a great way to rest the mind and renew the body.

For people who do not have a regular exercise routine or who haven't exercised in a long time, we recommend that you check with your physician, and if appropriate, begin with walking—in water or on land. The average walking program begins with fifteen to thirty minutes, once or twice a day. We don't ask participants to take their pulses, but suggest they walk slowly enough that they are not out of breath and can carry on a normal conversation. Usually, participants continue at the same level for three or four days. If they're not tired or sore afterwards, they increase the duration of their walk by five minutes. They increase their exercise by five minutes every three or four days until they are walking at least one and one-half hours per day. Most participants can achieve one and one-half hours per day within three to four weeks. Some eventually walk as much as three to four hours a day while they are with us. Exercise sessions might be divided into two or more periods of at least twenty to thirty minutes per session. Once you have reached your weight loss goals, one hour per day is a good idea to maintain your health.

Ricers who are limited by illness or orthopedic problems can begin their exercise program with as little as one to two minutes of exercise once or twice a day, and increase the duration of their exercise in one to two minute increments every week or so. It doesn't matter how long it takes to progress or how much you can walk in the first month. What matters is that you've begun, and over the next months you will see improvement. One participant with severe lung disease had to be taken by wheelchair from her hotel room to the bus, which carried her to the Rice House. After a week on the diet, we asked her to walk around her hotel room two to four times a day. A week later we increased the distance to 10 feet down the hall and back, then 20

> Exercise is a lifetime commitment. It is also a commitment to life. "The real miracle is not to walk on water or in the air. The real miracle is to walk on the earth."
>
> —*Thich Nhat Hanh*

Be cautious about hot tubs, steam rooms, or saunas while on the low-sodium levels (Phases One and Two) of the diet. These might cause you to be light-headed and/or faint. Once you increase your sodium to maintenance level (Phase Three) this should not be a problem.

feet and so on until she could walk from her room to the bus and beyond.

Patients who cannot walk can often do water walking, swimming, or pool exercises with a slow pace and progression similar to the walking program. If these sports don't appeal to you, try walking on a treadmill, Nordic tracking, elliptical trainers, bicycling, stair stepping, and sports like tennis. Again, check with your physician before beginning more vigorous exercise.

You might want to choose a secondary or seasonal activity if weather affects your exercise plan. Just commit to develop your own personal exercise prescription or plan what you think is realistic for you. For example, my NYC-born husband, Bob, doesn't like to break a sweat in North Carolina, so he is an elliptical trainer devotee; you needn't waste your time in trying to sell him on anything else. Whereas, I am the outdoor enthusiast and don't think a day is all it could be without walking the Eno River, or as fellow Ricers fondly know, "the trail." You also don't want to try to schedule something with me during my two hours of Pilates per week!

Consider weight training as well. Remember our muscle mass accounts for most of the calories we burn. Maintaining muscle mass really helps to keep your weight under control. So do some weight training two to three times a week in addition to your walk or swim, not as a replacement. We also recommend using an exercise trainer, at least initially. If you want to do more vigorous exercise, don't forget to check with your physician.

# START YOUR WALKING PROGRAM

As we mentioned previously, walking is a great way to begin a regular exercise program because it's one of the most convenient, rewarding, and fun activities, and helps people stick with this part of the *dieta*. The following are tips to help you get started on your own walking program.

## DETERMINING THE RIGHT DISTANCE

If you are just starting a walking program and uneasy about your endurance level, go to a track at a local school or college. On a track you can walk as much or as little as you want, and if you want to calculate your distance, most tracks are one-quarter of a mile around (in circumference), so four trips around the track equal a mile. Another plus: state-of-the-art track surfaces are usually easier on your joints than concrete or pavements. But don't get hung up on how much distance you cover; focus on the duration of time.

Using time as your measurement, an "out and back" walk is an easy way to develop new walking routes and increase your exercise endurance. "Out and back" simply means that you walk from a certain point, say your house, and then when you feel that you have gone halfway, you turn around and come back.

# WORDS TO PONDER AS YOU WALK

Dr. Francis Neelon is one of the most important—and most beloved—physicians who guides, advises, and supports participants during their stay at the Rice Diet Program. Dr. Neelon is also known for his love affair with the English language, whether in the form of poetry or prose. Over the years, he has collected the following selection of quotes from some of his favorite writings.

*Of all exercises walking is the best.*—Thomas Jefferson

*Before supper take a little walk, after supper do the same.*—Erasmus

*Perhaps the truth depends on a walk around the lake.*—Wallace Stevens

*A vigorous five-mile walk will do more good for an unhappy but otherwise healthy adult than all the medicine and psychology in the world.*
—Paul Dudley White

*Take a two-mile walk every morning before breakfast.*—Harry Truman (advice on how to live to be eighty on his eightieth birthday)

*The sum of the whole is this: walk and be happy; walk and be healthy. The best way to lengthen out our days is to walk steadily and with a purpose.*
—Charles Dickens

*If you are seeking creative ideas, go out walking. Angels whisper to a man when he goes for a walk.*—Raymond Inmon

*Above all—do not forget to walk. Everyday I walk myself into well-being and walk away from every illness. I have walked myself into my best thoughts and know of no thought so burdensome that I cannot walk myself out of it.*
—Buddha

# LONG, SLOW DISTANCE

We have always advocated working up to, then walking long, slow distances (LSD). It's easier on the joints. We also advocate walking at least one hour a day for several reasons. First, you get all the health benefits. Second, you burn enough calories to be 20 to 40 pounds lighter than if you didn't walk an hour daily after one year. And, third, but perhaps most important, walking an hour a day means you have to take an hour a day for yourself. Not taking time for ourselves is the major reason we don't take better care of ourselves. And not taking time for ourselves is a major cause of stress in our lives and stress is a major reason for unhealthy behavior. The only reason for not walking an hour a day is that we are using some of that time for meditation, tai chi, or yoga. Of course, it would be better to add those activities to our hour walk and take more than an hour a day for ourselves.

Walking outdoors is best. Walking silently with someone else works fine, too. You get the health benefits, burn the calories, and get time with yourself. If you prefer exercising on a machine while watching TV, reading, or listening to your iPod or Walkman, then take some other opportunity for quiet time to be with yourself that day.

Making the time for exercise every day is an important step to becoming truly mindful in your life. If you feel you don't really have one hour, first ask yourself if that makes any sense. In an average daily schedule, you need one hour for exercise and around eight hours for sleep. That still leaves fifteen hours for everything else. If you don't want to take one hour for exercise, take less, but do some exercise daily.

Regardless of how you make time for yourself—through meditation, yoga, tai chi, or more standard forms of exercise—the point is to prioritize this time. Think about yourself and how you want to live. How you live is a choice and a commitment. "But, Doctor," you say, "I'll wind up taking an hour and a half or even two hours a day

# CALORIES BURNED DURING A WALK AT 2 TO 3 MPH SPEED

| Weight | Calories/Mile | Weight | Calories/Mile | Weight | Calories/Mile |
|---|---|---|---|---|---|
| 100 | 69 | 170 | 119 | 230 | 162 |
| 110 | 75 | 180 | 126 | 240 | 168 |
| 120 | 82 | 190 | 131 | 250 | 174 |
| 130 | 94 | 200 | 140 | 260 | 180 |
| 140 | 100 | 210 | 149 | 270 | 189 |
| 150 | 106 | 220 | 156 | 275 | 193 |

for myself." Great! The more seriously you take this time commitment for yourself, the greater your chances of achieving and maintaining your desired weight and health, and truly being available to be who you want to be for yourself, others, and the world.

Your goal now is to figure out how you can rest so that you can be mindful—not just of your eating but of yourself and the life you want for yourself. In a state of peace, you are more likely to be able to envision an ideal life—one in which you lose weight, achieve your weight goal, attain better health, and live fully. Be in the moment. So where does the path to true restfulness lead? To a place where your new *dieta* is effortless because you are at one with it, at peace. Here's to us all creating and prioritizing more sacred time for ourselves, which will enhance the actualization of our dreams and goals.

# CHAPTER SIX

# LIVING THE DIET

*We want to overcome a habit, such as smoking, for the health of our body and mind. When we begin the practice, our habit energy is still stronger than our mindfulness, so we don't expect to stop smoking overnight. We have only to know that we are smoking when we are smoking. As we continue to practice, looking deeply and seeing the effects that smoking has on our body, mind, family, and community, we become determined to stop. It is not easy, but the practice of mindfulness helps us to see the desire and the effects clearly, and eventually we will find a way to stop. "The seventh miracle is transformation."*

—THICH NHAT HANH, *SEVEN MIRACLES OF MINDFULNESS*

I t's true. The diet takes work and energy—to think about the foods, plan your meals, shop, and remember to exercise and make time for yourself. But soon, this "new way of living" will feel more natural and will require less energy. We promise! As you grow accustomed to the foods, the portion sizes, and the way your body responds to your new way of eating, you will need to think about your foods less frequently, plan with less effort, and all in all, expend less energy *doing* the diet. You will simply *live* the diet. The most significant power of this *dieta* is that it becomes easier as you become conscious that it is what you are *choosing* to do with your life, not one more thing on your "have-to-do" list. If a diet is nothing but a chore, you're doomed to failure. But if you can embrace the *dieta*, it naturally fuels your desire to manifest your dreams and goals. You're co-creating your desired weight and life.

You have plenty of tools to help you tailor the diet so it works best for you and helps you find success in this moment, and in the next moment. What follows is a gathering of practical lists and guidelines to facilitate more and more of these successful moments, until you have a firm foundation of habits and tools that will equip and inspire you to live the program—now and forever.

# FIND YOUR DIET

Although we've offered a step by step approach to doing the diet, you can really do the diet in an infinite number of ways. It comes down to a question of what works best for you. As we often say to Ricers, "Go ahead and eat that chocolate bar, just do so mindfully." Are we advocating eating chocolate bars? Of course not. But we are also telling you loud and clear, "Do not waste your time on judging yourself and don't waste your energy on striving to do everything 'right.' " What's right is what's right for you. If you figure out what helps you to eat in a nutritious, mindful way, choosing foods that inspire you to lose weight and maintain it, then you have chosen what's "right" for you. It's that simple.

In the same breath we should also share that those who we've seen *keep their palate clean of sodium and refined foods until they reach their health goals* do better at actually meeting their goals and keeping them long-term. A famous 12-Step slogan is "if you don't want to fall down, don't go in slippery places!"

Everybody has their own way of living the diet long-term. One participant told us that he enjoys eating out with his new girlfriend. On Friday nights they go out for sushi and on Saturday nights they go to their favorite Italian restaurant on Mulberry Street in New York City's Little Italy. He eats whatever he wants—if he wants salami, he eats salami; if he wants a Florentine bistecca, he eats his steak; if he wants tiramisu, he enjoys a couple of bites of the puffy, creamy pastry. We looked at him in surprise, because he had clearly not regained any of the weight he had lost while at the Program.

"Well how do you do it?" we asked.

"On Monday, I eat rice and fruit. On Tuesday, Wednesday, and Thursday, I add vegetables. It's my new girlfriend. As long as I stick with one woman, I won't be in trouble. But if I were taking two or three women out twice a week, then I'd be back in trouble in no time! Committing to one good woman and the Rice Diet Program has made my life great!"

Whatever it takes, right?

This participant has found a way to tailor the diet to suit him. He eats what he wants, but he does it in a structured, mindful way. So let's figure out how to find *your* diet.

Many participants with eating addictions say that eating the Rice Diet is not as difficult as they thought it would be because its simplicity keeps them far from the binge or trigger foods that they want to avoid until they are closer to where they want to get with their weight and health improvements. Trust your feelings. If, after moving from Phase One to Phase Two, you begin to snack or eat more, return to one day of the Basic Rice Diet. Once clear, decide whether you want to return to Phase One or continue with Two for another week. Your *dieta* choice is your responsibility to intend, declare, plan, and enjoy; then reassess what works, what doesn't, and what next. It is a *dieta* for life, not a "diet" that you go on and off.

We have designed the Rice Diet to be 800 to 1,200 calories per day, but you can tailor the diet (both the foods and the number of calories) to suit your needs. In other words, if you have reached your weight loss goals, have integrated mind-body activities and exercise, and you feel good, then you can make some 200 calorie additions (see page 40 in Chapter 2 for approximate calories and servings in the different food groups). Here are some choices to consider:

• **You can increase the number of servings of fresh fruits and vegetables.** Since these are very low in fat and sodium and full of antioxidant-rich nutrients, they are the safest and healthiest addition.

• **You can eat fish more than once each week.** This is one of the healthier ways to enjoy a couple of hundred extra calories. In fact, fish is far higher in omega-3 fatty acids than any other food. If you have a history of heart disease or arthritis, it would probably be the healthiest addition to choose.

• **You can use more food accents such as olive oil, nuts, and seeds.** Be sure to refresh your memory on fatty-food portion sizes: 1 teaspoon of oil equals 1 to 2 tablespoons of nuts or seeds equals 45 calories. Obviously, the higher fat and calorie foods tend to be easier to overeat, in which case you might regret adding them later. Just be sure to stay mindful. Journalize. If eating today's intended 2 table-spoons of walnuts becomes a munchathon while you're watching a good movie and de-stressing later that night, it's time to reassess your food choices and select foods that do not inspire bingeing.

• **You can add dairy products** if you did not notice "detox" or aller-gic responses when you "cleaned out" with soy milk rather than cow's milk. You may have noticed less congestion, sluggishness, and fatigue when on a vegetarian diet in Phase One, so you may choose to stick with soy or grain milks instead of cow's milk. Calcium-fortified soy milk is probably the healthiest choice; nonfat yogurt, skim milk, ½ percent dry curd cottage cheese (the low-sodium type, with yogurt added to improve the texture) are also good choices. You can enjoy small (1 to 2 tablespoons) amounts of grated Parmesan, or other cheeses a couple of times per week. Again, be mindful of quantity, as salty, flavorful foods like cheese can trigger many to overeat. Two tablespoons of freshly grated Parmesan cheese contains only 46 calories, but if you go back for a few big hunks (4 ounces) you've exceeded your addition challenge times ten. A word of caution: many find cheese to be a very slippery slope.

• **You can add more foods to your diet such as lean meat or poultry** (if you aren't a heart patient); preferably the leaner cuts, wild game, or one to two eggs per week.

• **You can structure your eating plan** using the total calories per week instead of the daily total, and mix and match your foods more creatively. For example, if like the person above, you enjoy eating out with no rules, then do so, and then cut back on calories the rest of the week by relying on the Basic Rice Diet for a Monday reality check! (Remember, there is an easy way to keep track of calories; consult the portion control table on page 40 in Chapter 2.) Keep your food record (see pages 128–129 for more information) so you will realize if and when your old food habits are taking over your brain!

How you do the diet is up to you. That's why it's so livable—it's your diet.

# YOUR JOURNAL

We have found that most Ricers benefit greatly from keeping a daily journal, especially in the first few months of getting accustomed to the Rice Diet and their new *dieta*. Use the upcoming journal worksheet as a way to monitor your ongoing progress and pitfalls, or shall we say learning opportunities! It can help you increase both your self-awareness and your responsibility for what you are eating and doing each day. Essentially, you will be recording your:

• **daily weight**

• **goals for that day in terms of nutrition and calories**

• **meal intake**

• **exercise routine**

• **mindfulness time**

• **progress in terms of weight lost, gained, or maintained**

• **blood pressure and blood sugars (document these if you have had these elevated in the past)**

# ACTUAL FOOD INTAKE AND GOALS

Keeping a record of your food, exercise, and feelings is one of the most respected predictors of who loses weight and keeps it off.

Tracking your daily food intake on these pages offers a huge break-through for many who eat more than they are aware of. Feel free to copy these pages for ongoing use, or you may prefer to order your *Personal Journal for Health* from the Rice Diet Store (www.rice dietstore.com) for monthly or quarterly encouragement. (See Appendix B for further information.) Be sure to include all foods that you eat, even if they are outside your goal intake. Don't beat yourself up. Don't judge yourself. Simply be honest and kind.

Your total intake will be the total number of starches, vegetables, fruits, dairy, protein, and fat based on the meal plans in this chapter as well as in the recipe section. We also recommend that you keep track of each food group consumed at breakfast and lunch so you can adjust dinner intake if you need to. If you've recorded your meal plan goals on the worksheet as well, you will have an easier time visualizing the amount of food you intend to eat. Here is the key to the abbreviations used:

S=starches    V=vegetables    D=dairy    FR=fruit
P=protein*    F=fat
*Remember, in Phase One, you will not be eating protein in the form of fish, chicken, or lean meat.

You may find that the simple act of documenting everything you eat or drink inspires mindful eating. If numbers and details will only discourage you, then please only document your intake. (See Food Journal on page 126.) Others may be inspired further by tracking their calories, fat, and sodium intakes, and educating themselves on the specifics of nutrition. (See Appendix B for how to obtain a small *T-Factor* book, if you prefer a pocket-sized reference for such dietary details. For a larger data bank of foods and their nutritional components you can go to the USDA's food data bank at www .nal.usda.gov/fnic/foodcomp.)

# EXERCISE

Track your physical activity on a daily basis. We recommend a total goal of five to seven hours of walking per week. In addition to cardiovascular exercise, we recommend strength training for thirty to forty minutes twice a week (i.e., see page 108 for more information), stretching on a daily basis, and thirty minutes of mind-body relaxation or meditation daily. And think of this: tai chi and yoga can accomplish stretching, strength training, and meditation goals all at once!

# WEIGHING YOURSELF

Keep track of how you are doing by weighing yourself each and every day—in the morning after going to the bathroom. We believe checking the scale each day helps you to remember that you've made your weight loss a priority. Just as you brush your teeth daily in order to take care of your teeth, weigh yourself daily. It is a concrete way of caring for yourself and staying mindful of your attention and intention for this important aspect of your life. Though you weigh every day, you only examine your journal and check how you're doing once a week. You will find that there is one day (usually Thursday or Friday) when you weigh the least for the week. If you're not losing week to week, review your diet and exercise program. If you're doing what you've intended to, continue. This is a race you cannot lose. You will win unless you drop out.

# YOUR PERSONAL NOTES

We have found that writing down your daily thoughts and feelings in the "Personal Notes" section is a helpful, often elucidating experience that enriches your mindfulness and helps your overall success on the Rice Diet. Why record your feelings? There are many reasons: to keep your awareness on yourself and your dreams; to heal or manage the conditions that inspired your weight problem, which often percolate up to consciousness when one discontinues a "drug of choice"; to take a closer look at your emotional issues; to record your inner spiritual journey; to record biologic or physiologic changes as they occur. This is your place to write about whatever you want—the diet, the day, or life in general. If you get in touch with what you truly desire from life, if you have a concrete, specific vision of the future that you want, then you will be more successful in actualizing that future by standing in the commitment to become conscious of the circumstances leading to your overweight. Many Ricers have said how invaluable their journal entries were months and years later, helping them renew their long-term commitments, while reminding themselves how great they felt after only one to two weeks on the diet.

Intention, declaration, and action are all key pieces to establishing and realizing our goals and dreams. We don't achieve greatness, the potential of who we are here to be, by thinking small, or using vague language. We coach our participants at the Rice Diet Program to say what they mean and mean what they say; to discover and stay in the truth that is theirs. For example, instead of saying: "I *wish* I could lose *some* weight and have my joints hurt *less*, but *my arthritis* is *inherited* from my Mama and my Daddy's side of the family are all heavy. *We're just big people* who like food." Whew! This person isn't going anywhere fast, much less harnessing all the power she has to participate in her healing. She is still *wishing* upon a star that she could someday lose *some* (she has no vision for her desired weight) weight and have her joints hurt (some unknown degree) *less.* She's using vernacular that helps her accept her arthritis and she's clinging to the false beliefs that she is also helpless in the face of her genetic propensity for arthritis and obesity. She has given her power over to her genes and joined a club that is "just big and likes food." As long as she chooses to operate with these beliefs, the neurological pathways that help create these responses will continue to deepen, and she'll continue to drown her misery in food. The good news is that she can choose to perceive things differently, in this moment, and in the next, and in the next.

This same woman can choose to open herself to the possibility that what she thinks and says and journals and does can improve her chances of succeeding with her quest to reduce her weight and pain. She can commit to meditating (joining a class or buying a Thich Nhat Hanh or Jon Kabat-Zinn meditation tape), journalizing, and joining a group to increase her awareness of what she wants: her goals, her words, and her actions. As she readies herself via these paths (among many more) she can more fruitfully intend and declare: "I choose this *dieta* to provide the path that I will follow to reach my weight goal of 128 pounds, by January 9. I choose to activate the healing power within me to alleviate the arthritis pain by my commitment to practice yoga or tai chi at least fifteen minutes daily (or another gentle stretching discipline), swim or do water aerobics for one hour three times per week, walk at least three hours per week, and practice my meditation and journalizing daily fifteen to sixty minutes."

We may still have doubts about our ability to achieve our goals, so declaring them is often a difficult step. However, you can choose to be the little engine that could rather than couldn't. There is an incredible amount of quantum physics research showing that our beliefs create our reality far more than we ever imagined. One of the reasons why so many 12-Step program participants have been successful is that they repeat powerful affirmations to reinforce their new beliefs about themselves. Instead of continuing with the same beliefs and thought processes and actions, and expecting different results, they express the intention to "act as if . . ." So in other words, if you have intended and declared that you are committed to this phenomenal *dieta*, and wake up and don't feel like getting out of bed to do your yoga, instead of ruminating on how "this is what I always do, have great goals and then do what I've always done—not follow through with them," remind yourself "I can choose to perceive things differently and I choose to 'act as if' this is what I most want to do with my morning. I can choose to co-create the weight, health, and life I desire, and I choose to follow my game plan."

A huge part of being successful with this *dieta*, or frankly anything, is developing a life vision, a dream beyond what society and others have expected of you, a specific plan for what you truly want.

Take a half hour or so alone with a journal, close your eyes, take a few deep breaths, and relax more with each exhalation. Then gently ask yourself, "If I were guaranteed of not failing, what are three dreams that I would like to realize in my lifetime?" Regardless of how crazy or surprising the thoughts that surface may be, write them down. Relinquish your judgment and go with what comes up from this question. You may want to periodically touch base with your inner self. Many have not spoken to the captain of their ship in years!

Once our intention and declaration are aligned, moving mountainous habits is much easier. As one of my favorite body workers, Rodonna, recently said to me, "I never start on someone's back when they come in with back pain. I look at their body and see where they are holding (tension or blocked energy). When I address the source of the problem, it's a lot less work for both of us for the problem to release and heal." The same is true with healing weight issues or any other symptom of "dis-ease." Rest, reflect, release the root blockage or unrelinquished pain or source, renew, then do what you really have been wanting to do with your life. The next step is a tool to help you "do" this for the long haul.

# SAMPLE FOOD JOURNAL

# YOUR DIET PLAN (1200 CALORIE)

**Date 1/9**

**Today's Weight:** ____243____    **Blood Pressure/Other:** ____160/98____

| Serving Size | Food | Cals / Fat / Sodium | | |
|---|---|---|---|---|
| Breakfast | 1 c. oatmeal | 145 | 2 | 0 |
| | 3 prunes | 60 | 0 | 0 |
| | 1 c. skim milk | 90 | 0 | 120 |
| | 1 banana | 111 | 1 | 1 |
| | TOTAL | 405 | 3 | 121 |

S= **2**     V= **0**     FR= **3**     P= **0**     D= **1**     F= **0**

| | | | | |
|---|---|---|---|---|
| Lunch | 1 c. brown rice | 232 | 2 | 0 |
| | 1 c. steamed broccoli | 46 | 1 | 41 |
| | 1⅓ c. strawberries | 66 | 1 | 3 |
| | TOTAL | 344 | 4 | 44 |

S= **3**     V= **2**     FR= **1**     P= **0**     D= **0**     F= **0**

| | | | | |
|---|---|---|---|---|
| Dinner | 3 oz. cooked snapper | 109 | 2 | 48 |
| | 1½ c. potato | 240 | 0 | 13 |
| | 2 c. tossed salad | 40 | 0 | 71 |
| | ½ c. stewed tomatoes | 35 | 0 | 31 |
| | 1 c. fruit sorbet | 240 | 0 | 22 |
| | TOTAL | 664 | 2 | 185 |

S= **3**     V= **3**     FR= **4**     P= **3**     D= **0**     F= **0**

**TOTALS:** **S**tarch = 8       **V**egetables = 5       **FR**uit = 8

**P**rotein = 3       **D**airy = 1       **F**at = 0

Daily Total for Cals/Fat/Sodium          1,413      9          350

| Meal Plan Goals | Actual Intake | Differences (+/−) between Goals & Intake |
|---|---|---|
| S= 8 | 8 | _____ |
| V= 5 | 5 | _____ |
| FR= 3 | 8 | +5  (from fruit sorbet's 240 cals) |
| P= 3 | 3 | _____ |
| D= 1 | 1 | _____ |
| F= 0 | 0 | _____ |

| Daily Activity: | Goal | Actual |
|---|---|---|
| Cardiovascular | 60 mins. | 60 |
| Strength Training | 30 mins. 2 x weekly | 20 |
| Flexibility (stretching) | Daily | 60 |
| Mind/Body Relaxation | 30 mins. | 60 |

**Personal Notes:**

Today I attended the Journalizing class at the Rice Diet Program. I frankly wasn't expecting much from the experience but was amazed at what came up for me. When I asked myself where the last 50 pounds came from . . . I didn't know that I had the answer until I started writing about how my weight was protecting me from feeling my feelings. I was shocked to see that I was eating my feelings rather than feeling my feelings. My New Year's resolution is to journalize daily!

P.S. That fruit sorbet was no fat but those 240 calories were sure not as nutritious, satisfying, or filling as 4 cups of cold watermelon would have been.

# FOOD JOURNAL

## YOUR DIET PLAN

**Date** _____

**Today's Weight:** _____ **Blood Pressure/Other:** _____

| **Serving Size** | **Food** | **Cals / Fat / Sodium** |
|---|---|---|

Breakfast

**S=** \_\_\_  **V=** \_\_\_  **FR=** \_\_\_  **P=** \_\_\_  **D=** \_\_\_  **F=** \_\_\_

Lunch

**S=** \_\_\_  **V=** \_\_\_  **FR=** \_\_\_  **P=** \_\_\_  **D=** \_\_\_  **F=** \_\_\_

Dinner

**S=** \_\_\_  **V=** \_\_\_  **FR=** \_\_\_  **P=** \_\_\_  **D=** \_\_\_  **F=** \_\_\_

**TOTALS:** **S**tarch = \_\_\_  **V**egetables = \_\_\_  **FR**uit = \_\_\_

**P**rotein = \_\_\_  **D**airy = \_\_\_  **F**at = \_\_\_

Daily Total for Cals/Fat/Sodium  \_\_\_  \_\_\_  \_\_\_

| Meal Plan Goals | Actual Intake | Differences (+/−) between Goals & Intake |
|---|---|---|
| S= _____ | _____ | _____ |
| V= _____ | _____ | _____ |
| FR= _____ | _____ | _____ |
| P= _____ | _____ | _____ |
| D= _____ | _____ | _____ |
| F= _____ | _____ | _____ |

| Daily Activity: | Goal | Actual |
|---|---|---|
| Cardiovascular | 60 mins. | _____ |
| Strength Training | 30 mins. 2 x weekly | _____ |
| Flexibility (stretching) | Daily | _____ |
| Mind/Body Relaxation | 30 mins. | _____ |

**Personal Notes:**

_____

_____

_____

_____

_____

_____

_____

_____

_____

_____

_____

## INSPIRATIONAL CORNER

"I came to the Rice House because I hit rock bottom in that I was embarrassed to be seen in public, and avoided social obligations. Now that I am leaving the Rice House to go home, I was just thinking about how successful I have been on the program, and I am delighted to have lost 30 pounds in two months. Thanks for making my stay in Durham with the Rice program a most profitable experience."—D.F.

# FOCUSING ON FOOD LABELS

Food labels can provide you with a lot of information to help you make wise choices about what to eat. In general, the contents include the ingredients, serving size, calories, fat grams, saturated fat grams, percent of calories coming from fat, milligrams of cholesterol and sodium, grams of fiber, and kind and amount of additives (refined sugar, artificial sweeteners, preservatives, and colorings).

Take a look at how the ingredients are listed; they will appear in the order in which they are found in a product, by weight. For example, if sugar is the first ingredient listed, that means there is more sugar in the product than any other ingredient. Remember, it's in your best interest to choose foods that are made of whole, unadulterated ingredients that are naturally low in fat, sodium, and refined sugar.

You also want to pay attention to the serving size. Many packages declare the calorie count according to an unrealistically small serving size. For instance, some low-calorie cereals state ¾ to 1 cup as a serving size, whereas some high-calorie types (such as granolas) might state their serving size to be as small as ¼ cup! It might surprise a customer that a 15-ounce can of soup is considered to be three servings by some companies. So be aware that many products might contain more than one serving per container.

In addition to assessing the serving size and checking ingredients for sodium, refined sugars, and fat, evaluate the type of fat they use. As you may remember from Chapter 4, all fats contain saturated, monounsaturated, and polyunsaturated fatty acids. Saturated fat intake is the most respected predictor of high cholesterol. So reduce your intake of saturated fat–rich butterfat (butter, cheese, whole milk, cream sauces/soups), beef, pork, coconut, palm or palm kernel oil, and hydrogenated fats. Hydrogenated fats are oils that create smoother, creamier products with a longer shelf life. Unfortunately, these oils also contain more saturated and trans fats. The most commonly eaten hydrogenated fats include shortening, margarine, and most processed grain products (cookies, crackers, cereals, and breads), as well as spreads, dressings, and sauces.

Keep your oil consumption to 1 to 2 teaspoons of added oil per day, or 4 to 9 grams. This includes those oils added to processed or packaged foods—so read the fine print! For your 1 to 2 teaspoons of added oil per day, we highly recommend olive oil and canola oil. Canola oil has less saturated fats than any cooking oil we know. Other beneficial oils include walnut and toasted sesame seed oils for great flavoring of salads. Nuts and seeds are the ultimate source of fats if you can eat a teaspoon or two and stop before the munchies take over your mind.

Again, remember to note the milligrams (mg) of sodium listed in a product. This is of utmost importance since a product can advertise "no salt added," yet still contain other sodium-rich ingredients. Limit (or try to avoid if you're hypertensive) any products containing salt and anything with sodium in it—including monosodium glutamate (a flavor enhancer) or sodium benzoate (a preservative). Otherwise some added sodium in foods such as olives or capers is acceptable if those foods don't trigger you to want more and more salt. Remember, our goal is to consume between 500 and 1,000 milligrams of sodium per day.

# FOOD LABEL WORKSHEET

Product: _____

Ingredients: _____

Serving Size _____ Calories/Serving _____

Protein grams _____ Carbohydrate grams _____ Fat grams _____

$$\% \text{ of calories from fat} = \frac{\underline{\hspace{2cm}} \text{ grams fat} \times 9 \text{ calories/gram}}{\underline{\hspace{2cm}} \text{ total calories}} \times 100$$

% of calories coming from fat _____

List fat-rich ingredients _____

Is the fat saturated?_____ monounsaturated rich? _____

omega-3 rich? _____ omega-6 rich? _____

trans fats? _____ partially hydrogenated fats? _____

Does the product contain cholesterol? _____

Sodium mg _____ Naturally occurring or added salt? _____

Does it contain refined sugar?_____

Is it a significant source of fiber?_____

Highly recommend: _____

Conditionally recommend: _____

Alternatives: _____

Avoid, list reasons: _____

Product evaluation/comments: _____

# USING SPICES

When we talk about spices, we should talk about herbs and spices together. An herb is defined as a plant useful for its leaf, flower, stem, or root. Spices are the dried berries, seeds, or bark of certain trees and bushes, such as black pepper, cinnamon, nutmeg, and mustard. Herbs and spices enhance the flavors of foods, and add to the enjoyment of eating without much sodium and fat.

In the past, Dr. Kempner did not permit any use of herbs and spices while on the Rice Diet Program, although patients were permitted to use them freely once they returned home. Dr. Kempner thought that using flavor enhancers would act as an appetite stimulant. These days we use herbs and spices at the Rice House in the cooking of grains and vegetables and have not heard complaints that they have increased the participants' appetites. However, herbs and spices should be consumed with awareness.

After sufficient time on the Rice Diet, especially if you are doing the Basic Rice Diet weekly, your palate begins to change. You will notice that you require much less added flavoring and enjoy your food much more thoroughly. When many Americans eat today, they are not tasting the food, but the salt that is used to flavor it. One patient realized he didn't actually like shrimp, he only liked the cocktail

## TIP

Always taste the food item first, then season. Seasoning is a highly personalized thing, and not everyone likes the same flavors, but there are certain food/seasoning pairings that work well.

sauce! You may enjoy the following spices to enhance your food, not overwhelm it.

## SPICE IT UP

**Food to Be Seasoned and Suggested Seasonings**
Try one herb or spice at a time.

**Asparagus:** basil, chives, dill, nutmeg, sesame seeds, tarragon

**Beans (dried):** allspice, chili powder, coriander, cumin, garlic, marjoram, oregano, rosemary, sage, savory, tarragon, thyme

**Beans (green):** basil, bay leaves, dill, garlic, marjoram, rosemary, savory, tarragon

**Beans (lima):** basil, chives, dill, marjoram, sage, savory, tarragon

**Beets:** allspice, caraway seeds, chives, dill, ginger, horseradish

**Broccoli, Cauliflower, Cabbage, Brussels Sprouts (cruciferous vegetables):** basil, caraway seeds, curry powder, garlic, ginger, marjoram, oregano, tarragon, thyme

**Carrots:** caraway seeds, chives, cumin, ginger, marjoram, nutmeg, tarragon

**Corn:** chives, coriander, cumin, rosemary, sage, savory, thyme

**Eggplant:** allspice, basil, garlic, marjoram, oregano, sage, thyme

**Eggs:** chili powder, chives, cumin, curry powder, savory, tarragon

**Fish:** basil, bay leaves, chives, coriander, dill, nutmeg, sage, tarragon, lemon thyme, oregano

**Mushrooms:** basil, chives, dill, garlic, marjoram, oregano, rosemary, savory, tarragon

**Peas:** basil, chives, dill, marjoram, oregano, rosemary, tarragon

**Peppers (sweet):** basil, chives, coriander, garlic, Italian parsley, marjoram, oregano, thyme

**Potatoes:** bay leaves, caraway seeds, chives, coriander, curry powder, dill, garlic, mint, oregano, parsley, tarragon, thyme

**Rice:** chives, cumin, curry powder, garlic, sage, tarragon

**Shellfish:** basil, bay leaves, chervil, cloves, coriander, curry powder, dill, marjoram, oregano, tarragon, thyme

**Spinach:** basil, garlic, nutmeg, tarragon

**Squash (winter):** allspice, cinnamon, cloves, curry powder, ginger, mace, nutmeg

**Squash (yellow and zucchini):** basil, chives, coriander, dill, garlic, ginger, marjoram, oregano, rosemary, savory, tarragon

**Sweet Potatoes:** allspice, cinnamon, cloves, ginger, nutmeg

**Tomatoes:** basil, chives, coriander, dill, garlic, marjoram, oregano, rosemary, sage, savory, tarragon, thyme

**Turnips:** allspice, cinnamon, ginger, nutmeg

## TIP

Fresh herbs are always best and can be easily grown or obtained in the supermarket. If you have never grown herbs before, do yourself a favor. If you plant them outside in the spring you will enjoy them for months, and years if they are perennials (they will often double in size by next year). Cutting, preparing, or cooking with them freshly cut from your garden will connect you with the earth and the joys of eating fresh, whole, organically grown foods. You can also dry or freeze them for winter use. The flavor of the dried herb is twice as potent as the fresh, therefore in converting a recipe that has dried herbs, multiply by two (1 teaspoon dried parsley equals 2 teaspoons fresh parsley).

# EATING OUT

If you enjoy eating out at restaurants, you can do so and still stick to your Rice Diet program. Granted, low-fat, low-sodium, and low-sugar choices are not usually on the majority of restaurant menus, but the persistent diner can usually create them. You simply need to take some extra steps to plan ahead. The following tips may help you:

• **Contact the restaurant in advance** to ensure that the chef or kitchen is able to respond to your request for a dish that is low in fat and sodium. Be specific since the employee answering the phone may know very little about what low-sodium or low-fat means. For instance, ask if they have a fresh seafood, poultry, or vegetarian dish that can be prepared without added fat and salt. We don't suggest saying, "I am on a diet." Instead, explain that your doctor has recommended that you eat a specific way for a medical problem. Sometimes, people say that they are "allergic to salt." In certain countries it has been effective to acquire vegetarian meals by explaining that eating meat-free is part of one's religion or spiritual preference.

• **When you get to the restaurant, first ask if they have a heart-healthy menu.** If not, then ask your server for any suggestions about ordering a very simple fresh meal. A Ricer told me that she preferred asking them not to bring a menu (to tempt her), but instead to simply tell her what were the freshest fish and vegetables in the kitchen.

• **Don't be shy;** specify that your dish should be baked, broiled, or grilled without added sodium, and no more than one teaspoon of olive oil. You can even ask your waiter to "serve a 3 to 4 ounce portion, approximately the size of your palm, and go ahead and wrap the remainder to carry home" (for a great lunch the next day). Most of the more expensive restaurants will cook a very low-fat/sodium vegetarian or seafood entree for you upon request. The important thing to remember is that you don't know that a low-fat/sodium choice is out of the question until you ask for it! If you believe it is difficult or impossible, it likely will be. Approach this challenge with optimism: "When you expect the best, you often get it!"

• **If you are still having problems ordering,** scan the menu for dishes that use methods of preparation that are generally lowest in fat. Look for such words as steamed, broiled, roasted, grilled, and poached. Ask that the chef not add fat (except for a teaspoon of olive oil if you like) or sodium (including salt, broth, monosodium glutamate, and soy sauce) to your food, and to please flavor with wine, lemon, lime, garlic, and/or herbs. Avoid foods that are buttered, fried, creamed, in cream sauce, with gravy or hollandaise, au gratin, or pickled.

• **Remember to specify every item with low-fat/low-sodium instructions;** otherwise you might be served inappropriate side dishes. For instance, "May I please have fresh grilled tuna with a little olive oil and lemon but no added salt, a baked potato with no topping, and a tossed salad with olive oil and vinegar on the side?"

• **For buffet dining it is always smart to walk completely around the table before starting to make your choices.** By knowing all of the food choices, you are then equipped to make the lowest-fat/sodium, yet enjoyable, selections.

• **The best dessert is fresh fruit.** Other low-fat possibilities are ices and sherbet. Typically, however, the lower the fat content of frozen desserts, the higher the sugar and calories, so be careful. And another healthy option is to order the dessert of your choice to split, hopefully by four people!

Many restaurants now feature heart-healthy menus, but remember you get to take responsibility for what you eat; salud!

To order food in a Chinese restaurant without salt, MSG, or soy sauce, and stir fried in extra ginger, garlic, and wine, copy the Chinese characters below and present them to your waiter, if necessary. Then, if you choose, you can add freshly squeezed lemon juice and chili peppers. You will probably find that it is delicious without soy sauce added. This way you know what you are eating.

做饭不用油．盐．味精．也不用酱油．
Prepare food with no oil, salt, MSG, or soy sauce.

炒菜只用酒．姜和蒜．
Stir fry with wine and extra ginger and garlic.

•   •   •

These tools will not only make living the Rice Diet program doable and easier, they will enhance your overall experience. The journal especially is a tool that you can use again and again—not simply to keep track of your food intake and weight loss progress but to record your myriad thoughts and feelings during this transformative time in your life.

# CHAPTER SEVEN

# CREATE SUPPORT

*All the strong things in her heart came out in her body, that had been so tireless in serving generous emotions.*

—WILLA CATHER

# BUILDING YOUR COMMUNITY

Though you're the one who has to commit to the diet in order for it to work for you, getting support and encouragement from the people you live with is a very important component to living the *dieta*. Our community is integral to fostering transformation and supporting healthier behavior. Thich Nhat Hanh tells the story of a troubled teenager sent from an orphanage in England to Plum Village (his retreat center in France) for a retreat with other teenagers. No one in Plum Village knew the young woman's background or that she was troubled. As she began to follow the routine of her new community, practicing mindful breathing, mindful sitting, walking meditation, and mindful eating, she began to change from the inside out—though again, this change was not obvious to her new companions, as they had no basis for comparing her old self with her new self.

Shortly after her return to England, Thich Nhat Hanh received a letter from the orphanage saying that the young woman had returned to England utterly transformed. Not only was she happy and peaceful, but she had begun helping the other children. Her troublesome attitude and behavior, which she had been known for, had disappeared. In its place was a kind, peaceful, loving person. The directors of the orphanage were so excited by her change that they wanted to send twenty children the following summer. Thich Nhat Hanh had to refuse. His reasoning? In a community of twenty happy children, the one unhappy one had been transformed, but in a community of twenty unhappy children, the happy ones might be transformed.

This story echoes both the succor and the challenge found through community. In a new environment as a member of a new group, the young woman found the freedom to be who she truly was, rather than continuing to project her former, angry persona. She let go of negative behaviors because she was practicing inner peace and meditation, but also because she could let go of her former defensive, angry postures. Her new self was accepted, welcomed, and encouraged. Could she have made the same transformation back at the orphanage, surrounded by people who saw her in only one, mostly negative light? Possibly, but it's doubtful. And what of the twenty other unhappy children the orphanage wanted to send to Plum Village? It seems that Thich Nhat Hanh understood that their sheer number, already forming its own group, would outweigh the community already established at the Village.

When you join a group or participate in a relationship with someone else, you are naturally affected or changed by that experience. When the group is positive and has your best interest at heart, it can provide support, encouragement, love, understanding, and motivation for your personal endeavors. Such community or group experiences can be so impactful that they have the power to reshape a person's life, as we see every day at the Rice House. However, some groups or communities can also work against us, encouraging us into roles or boxes from which we find it difficult to escape.

Communities, in this way, can keep us from changing. One example of this comes to mind. A woman in her early fifties, F.N., came to the Rice Diet Clinic several times over the course of two and a half years (and several visits to the Rice Diet Program) and went from 332 pounds to 186 pounds. She continued to lose weight—some at the program and some at home—but she was constantly frustrated with her efforts. After her last visit, she returned home, where she lived with her mother, and put back on almost forty pounds.

When she returned to the Rice Diet Program for another visit, she explained to us why she thought she had gained back weight. She said in frustration, "I have a very controlling mother, and she did not like it that I wanted to eat in a different way. She's overweight, too, and she was very uncomfortable with me cleaning out the cupboard and eating healthy foods. But most of all she was threatened by my new way of living. She gave me a hard time. But I'm back, and I'm determined to do it this time."

And she has. She has lost all of the weight she had regained and is continuing to lose weight. She is an absolute marvel! She explains her renewed success as she says, "I am spending much more time preparing for when I go home. I am going to find my own place. That will be painful, but it's a matter of saving my own life. I already feel more free. And I know I can do it. The Rice Diet has taught me that."

Although her former home community was a negative influence, the new community she found both at the Rice House and the new relationships she established at home have helped develop her sense of certainty and inner trust. Now, whenever the *dieta* feels difficult or tiring, she knows what to do. She either calls one of her fellow Ricers, sends an e-mail off to one of us at the Rice Clinic, or makes a walking date with one of her friends who she knows supports her.

## LESSONS FROM GEESE

1. As each bird flaps its wings, it creates an updraft for the bird following. By flying in a "V" formation, the whole flock adds 71 percent greater flying distance than if the bird flew alone.

Lesson: People who share a common direction and sense of community can get where they are going quicker and easier because they are traveling on the tailwind of one another.

2. Whenever a goose falls out of formation, it suddenly feels the drag and resistance of trying to fly alone, and quickly gets back into formation to take advantage of the "lifting power" of the bird immediately in front.

Lesson: If we have as much sense as a goose, we will stay in formation with those who are headed where we want to go (and be willing to accept their help as well as give our help to others).

3. When the lead goose gets tired, it rotates back into the formation and another goose flies to the point position.

Lesson: It pays to take turns doing the hard tasks and sharing leadership with people, as with geese, we are interdependent on each other.

4. The geese in formation honk from behind to encourage those up front to keep up their speed.

Lesson: We need to make sure our honking from behind is encouraging—and not something else.

5. When a goose gets sick, wounded, or shot down, two geese drop out of formation and follow it down to help and protect it. They stay with it until it is able to fly again or dies. Then they launch out on their own, with another formation, or catch up with the flock.

Lesson: If we have as much sense as geese, we, too, will stand by each other in difficult times as well as when we are strong.

To us, the idea of community is based on going outside oneself to share, to question, to offer and receive support, to encourage, and to feel part of something larger. A community can be your family, your relationship with your partner or best friend, a group you meet once a week to dine with, or a buddy with whom you walk for an hour each day. Creating community does not mean you have to join a formal group, but rather that you consciously choose to reach out to people who can support your *dieta* goals. As painful as it can be, sometimes participants choose to let go of friendships. As one woman explained, "One of my oldest girlfriends just kept questioning me. 'Aren't you done with that diet yet? Why do you need to lose weight?' She would go so far as sabotaging me by inviting me over to her house for dinner and covering her table with all this food—chips, dip, cake, cookies—you name it! She didn't want me to lose weight; it was that simple. So I don't see her as much. Am I sad? I used to think I was sad, but it's more disappointment that I feel. Who needs friends that don't want what's best for you?"

# DEVELOPING SUPPORT GROUPS AT HOME

At the Rice Diet Program, a feeling of community occurs naturally among participants because they spend much of their day with other people who have common goals. Group discussions provide a structured, safe environment that facilitates a sense of community and provides a time for participants to discover and recognize their own inner guidance.

Group discussions are for sharing feelings and experiences instead of learning or dispensing facts. They are definitely not for "fixing" other participants. The guidelines may seem a bit serious, even exaggerated, but we have been a part of many such groups over the years and have witnessed just how emotionally charged people become when they begin to change their lives: they feel vulnerable, they get angry, they begin to feel feelings that have long been held at bay. So if you decide to form your own support group, keep in mind the following guidelines:

1. **Everything said and done in a support group is confidential. Confidentiality is your responsibility.**

2. **The purpose of the group is to share your feelings and experiences.**

3. **All feelings are good.**

4. **Listen; everyone needs to feel they are being heard.**

5. Seek to understand, as well as to be understood.

6. Make a commitment to be there.

7. Don't interrupt.

8. Do not talk for others or interpret what they say.

9. Do not talk about anyone who is not in the room.

10. Speak in the first person by using "I" statements.

11. Do a hard thing every day—*Grow!*

# OTHER FORMS OF OUTREACH

At the Rice House, the community plays an important role in helping people get comfortable with the diet, which in turn helps prepare them for living the *dieta* once they leave. And although the Rice Diet Program welcomes you with open arms, it is not necessary for you to come here in order to benefit from the concept of community. Here are other ways you can create support and community:

• **Contact the Rice Diet Program** through our Web site (www. ricediet.com), become a member, and form relationships with other Ricers.

• **Join the Rice Diet Program's electronic Message Board,** which is a self-moderating, free forum for those trying to lose and maintain weight at home. (You can read posts without registering at our Web site, but you must register in order to post your comments, thoughts, and ideas.) On this forum, you will read questions and comments about different phases of this diet. The staff of the Rice Diet Program monitors this forum daily and tries to answer as many questions as possible.

• **Join a 12-Step Group.** 12-Step groups of many kinds evolved out of Alcoholics Anonymous (AA), a group started by Bill Wilson. The therapeutic healing potential for numerous other addictions have evolved out of AA, including Overeaters Anonymous (OA), Adult Children of Alcoholics Anonymous (ACOA), and Smokers Anonymous (SA), to name a few. As with all of life's opportunities, it is to our advantage to enter into these groups with an open heart and mind, while practicing discernment. Overall, their success rate is unsurpassed by any other healing groups we know that are free and available to everyone, everywhere.

Many clubs may offer something to do with your time, entertainment, food, or access to a sport, but becoming conscious of who we spend our time with is of utmost importance. Which do you think is more empowering and healing: to hang out with people who are drinking alcohol, smoking cigarettes, and gossiping about one another; or to connect with a club or group that offers exercise classes, team sports, health-conscious potlucks, and renewal healing conferences and opportunities? We are not only what we eat, we become (to a degree) who we associate with. The power of honest communication in a community of similarly focused persons has phenomenal potential to heal and promote our dreams and goals.

• **If you belong to a church, investigate community groups or events** that are focused on healing or sharing, or consider starting one. Aqueduct Retreat Center is a Christian retreat center nestled atop a hill south of Chapel Hill, North Carolina. It is a community that has fueled and supported every major life decision and healing I (Kitty) have experienced in the last two decades. After numerous other healings experienced there, I began to understand the incredible power within us all to heal, and the importance of prioritizing rest, reflection, and renewal to maximize this potential to participate in our own full healing. Healing the problem at its source is better than spending a lifetime and a huge financial investment in medicines and surgery battling the symptoms.

• **Join a gym and accomplish two feats at once: exercise and community!** Again, shop around, interview the trainers, research which gym or spa near you has the greatest variety of services that will serve your needs. Some spas offer free yoga, so investigate them before joining.

• **Find a walking partner and schedule your walks a few times a week.** When demands in life try to invade your exercise time, practice this response: "I'd really love to, but I have a previous appointment at that time." You do not have to announce or explain that you scheduled this important appointment with yourself!

# SPIRITUAL HEALING AND THE ROLE OF RELIGION

Many people may not find their spirituality in a traditional religious setting, but rather in other situations and other places. Their strength may come from their friendships, their family, a hobby, pet, or other source of support. These may be sufficient for the person to live a satisfying life and overcome difficult life problems, including powerful addictions. If these are not sufficient—and they are not enough for many people—then some may seek the necessary strength from religious sources. For thousands of years, religion has been a source of comfort and healing for people who are wounded by the "slings and arrows of outrageous fortune." And while religion, when devoid of love, may be used for destructive purposes, the deepest wounds that people experience are often rooted in inner spiritual struggles—evidenced by a deep void inside that nothing seems to fill (not alcohol, not drugs, not wealth, not fame, not food). And yet, complete healing may not be achievable without addressing this void head on.

Many find this healing in religion and in the community aspects of religion. Indeed, research has begun to examine how religious beliefs and practices can impact people's health. Dr. Harold Koenig, a Duke University psychiatrist, is one of the top researchers on health benefits of a religious discipline and makes the subject very approachable in his many books and for our Rice Diet community. Literally hundreds of studies have shown that devout religious practices and active involvement in a faith community is associated with better mental health, better physical health, and less addiction to alcohol, drugs, and other powerful factors that can take control of a person's life. This research has shown that religiously involved people—those who pray, read religious scriptures, serve in a church, synagogue, or mosque, and/or perform altruistic activities that involve doing good for others and sacrificing one's own comfort— experience greater well-being, happiness, and satisfaction in life. They have lower blood pressure, stronger immune systems, healthier cardiovascular systems, and live longer than those who are not involved in such religious activities. This is usually not intended, and may be a natural "side-effect" of a spiritually devout life; the Christian world calls this the "fruit of the Holy Spirit." It is especially when religiously inspired people get their preoccupations and obsessive thoughts off themselves and open their heart and mind to others that the "benefits" of religious faith begin to emerge, and it is then that the person's sense of purpose and meaning in life begins to blossom. Whether you have a religious commitment or not, a spiritual discipline involving regular meditation practice has been shown to lower blood pressure and heart rate, and would prove beneficial in lowering stress and only enhance your weight loss.

# LOOKING INWARD

You are going to succeed with this diet just as you would with any diet in the short run. Your top priorities are losing weight and taking care of yourself. Now that we've given you the mechanics of the program, it's time to take a look inward and look at any other habits, patterns of behavior, or emotional issues that may be getting in the way of permanent change. In the last chapter, you began this process of looking inward when you made time for yourself and began becoming more aware of your thoughts. Often, the peace and clarity of mind that follows mind-body activities such as meditation, yoga, tai chi, or traditional exercise, is enough to keep your commitment to the diet unimpeded. However, some of us may need a little more work with our "stuff" in order to let go of unhelpful beliefs, habits, or unhealthy reactions to stressors.

The main reason that people have difficulty maintaining their program is their priorities change. Dr. Eugene Stead, one of Dr. Rosati's mentors, said the reason people are thin is because day in and day out they prefer to be thin. He followed that with the reason people are overweight is because day in and day out they prefer to be overweight. Although he sounded a little harsh, he was right. He was talking about priorities. If you feel pulled back into old, weight-gaining habits, then something must be replacing your conscious decision and commitment to lose weight and take care of yourself. Remember F.N., mentioned previously? Despite her consistent success over the years, she lapsed because she subconsciously decided her mother's overbearing personality needed to be mollified.

We have found that most of the participants who come to the Rice Diet Program have been taking care of everything and everyone but themselves. They take care of their partners, their children, their parents, their friends, their businesses: anything but themselves. We have heard patients say over and over again, "I've never really taken any time for myself before." Taking care of anything but yourself is a habit—and one that is not helpful to you or to others.

So why do your priorities change back from your new *dieta* on the Rice Diet to your old *dieta*? The three main reasons are (1) it's a habit, (2) stress, and (3) the deadly combination of habit and stress. So we have to concentrate on how to overcome habit and eliminate or reduce stress or reduce its impact.

Becoming mindful through meditation, yoga, tai chi, and exercise are wonderful ways to snap yourself back into the priorities of your Rice *dieta*. Reaching out for support and encouragement in your community are also crucial ways to maintain your focus and dedication to taking care of yourself. We also encourage Ricers to participate in individual, couples, and group therapy as appropriate and when possible. With such emotional support, your own point of view, thoughts, feelings, and experiences all become much more clear and therefore easier to manage. For instance, according to Thich Nhat Hanh, if your wife or husband says something that hurts you, you can say, "Darling, what you just said hurt me a lot and I would like to meet with you next week to talk about it." When the time for the talk comes, a referee (read couples counselor) may be helpful to mediate; or, the timing may be such that you can discuss it and resolve the issue without hurting each other further with words, or hurting yourself by numbing out with binge foods.

If you continue to play the tape in your head that repeats what your mother may have told you at an early age, "that you are too fat and lazy, and will never do anything about it," you may very well believe that it is true and then continue to act accordingly. Physicists have shown that the neurons sending such repetitious messages in our brain get stuck in reproducing such false beliefs and make it unlikely to change. Unless you are committed to a conscious pursuit of real truth, you will continue to reproduce old, inaccurate beliefs that reinforce results. The good news is that they have also proven that when fresh insights and reflections inspire a new perspective, these new beliefs can replace the old beliefs that have gotten in our way, that have unconsciously fueled unhealthy responses—like overeating.

The majority of participants who come to the Rice Diet Program come to lose weight, but the reasons behind how they became overweight vary greatly. Some people are overweight because they frequent fast-food sources, snack excessively, eat late, or drink alcohol or sugared beverages. The bottom line is that they are eating more in calories than they are expending in energy.

You can call this problem by many names: overeating, dysregulated eating, a habit, or an addiction. Regardless of what you call it, the treatment is the same. As we said in the beginning, you can treat it with a traditional psychological model. For example, you may be helped by discussing your past feelings of shame with a therapist because you were harshly judged as a child, examining how you chose food to comfort yourself, and have continued to do so regularly, re-creating a reality that is really not helpful, such as eating every time your feelings are hurt. A good therapist may be very helpful in leading you to better understand the root of your pain, and can help you process and heal this knee-jerk, old habit driven reaction.

The treatment of weight loss, an overeating disorder, dysregulated eating, or an overeating addiction is the same, and at the same time different for everyone. There are many paths that lead to healing. We will not spend a lot of time discussing and debating the importance and various categorizations of why and how the overeating occurred in your life. Rather, we want you to focus on developing your strategy for healing.

Thousands of people have come to the Rice Diet Program who have connected to and have transformed their lives via many different paths and practitioners: some have their epiphany while writing in their journals in their room late at night; some while sitting in Dr. Rosati's meditation classes; some have their *aha* moment with Jeff Georgi, our therapist, as he explains the intricacies of how the brain reacts differently in an addict; some have a heart and mind fusion when Dr. Neelon reads poetry while at the same time demystifying medicine; and some have made the diet work for them by swapping practical recipes and diet strategies with Rachelle, our dietitian, and other Ricers while walking Duke Gardens on Thursday afternoons. The common ingredient is all the people on the Rice Diet who succeed make time for themselves to look within, to explore who they really are and what they want to do with their health and life, and they continue to connect to this inner self in order to maintain the diet and live life fully.

Regardless of the origin of an overeating problem, it is possible for you to create a new belief that is empowering, transforming, and feels like truth to you. Any overeater can choose to go for a nice, slow walk, meditate, or practice yoga, with the intention of reflecting on her belief about her mother's judgment of her supposed overweight, lazy, and hopeless nature. She might experience hurt feelings, particularly shame, tears could follow, then possibly anger, resentment, rage, then likely intense feelings of hunger. If this person were near her refrigerator or favorite bakery, the experience could return to its old, familiar loop, and she might medicate the emotional pain with copious amounts of refined sugar, which would offer immediate, yet short-lived relief. She will have reinforced her old behaviors, and she will react even faster next time. Her binge would soon lead to a desire for another sugar rush, and possibly two or three more. Nausea and stomach upset would follow, along with shame and hopelessness and then she'd return home to spread the blame around, be short-tempered with the children, and verbally abusive or withdrawn from her spouse—whew! So much for improved digestion and peace on earth!

The mind-boggling truth is that the woman in our example made a choice, albeit an unconscious one. She didn't simply turn to sugary food to assuage her negative feelings; she *chose* to turn to food, acting out of her ingrained neurological wiring. Choosing food as a reaction to stress is quite often an unconscious choice. This is not a blame thing—it's a brain thing! It's also an invitation to open yourself to paths that have helped thousands of others become increasingly more conscious of what they are thinking, feeling, and thus doing.

It is a common choice in developed nations to consume processed foods when we are in emotional pain or stressed; we have probably all laughed at some comedy depicting this human response. The truth is not that you are fat, lazy, and hopeless. The truth is that you are reacting to the pain of your long-held belief that you are fat, lazy, and hopeless, and you can choose to believe otherwise, and to respond to stress with your whole brain engaged rather than the primitive base, the amygdala.

Changing our perspective starts with a commitment. Dr. Jerry Jampolsky's book, *Love Is Letting Go of Fear* (Celestial Arts, 2004), is one of the most profound books ever written on this subject. He states that "we can choose to perceive things differently." This simple truth is a profound gift and tool for stopping the insanity in our lives. If insanity is defined as doing the same thing over and over, but expecting different results, then we are acting insane when we continue to overeat calories, sodium, or in general undermine our health and lives. However, when we take time for ourselves, we take the first step in choosing to perceive ourselves differently, believe in our potential and power, and ultimately shift our paradigm for living.

There is hope for healing the overeating disorder and addictions in general. Forty-three percent of Rice Diet participants maintained their weight loss or had lost more weight at home six years after leaving the program. Many people commit to choosing to perceive things differently and succeed at doing so. When my eight-year-old son is frustrated because of his belief that he can't do something, one of my favorite mottos is, "Whether you think you can or think you can't, you're probably right!" I am not sharing this to guilt or blame anyone, but to empower, inspire, and renew your hope that now can be the moment you are willing to commit to your weight loss or healing or whatever life dream you have been waiting to embrace. It truly is *your* choice.

So the next time painful emotions begin to stir feelings, which may have previously fueled your overeating responses, choose to perceive things differently, believe that you are committed to achieving your goal weight or health parameter, and bring out any tool that you have been practicing to assist you. Rather than turn to the refrigerator, choose to walk—not to the nearest bakery—but on the trail. Remember to breathe. Make this moment meditative by consciously being grateful that you live in a time and place where changing your belief from "I'm hopeless," to "I choose to commit to create the life of my dreams, to fulfill and enjoy my potential" does not risk your life but gives it back to you!

# INSPIRATIONAL CORNER

J.R., or "The Grinch" to his friends, is just thirty years old, but he brings a lifetime of experience to his position as Head Chef at the Rice House. J.R.'s hard-working family has owned restaurants in Queens, New York, and Georgetown in Washington, D.C., since he was a boy. Working side by side with his brother, three sisters, and parents, he learned firsthand the secrets of preparing fresh, savory foods quickly. In fact, he earned the nickname "Chef Grinch" when he worked as what is known as a "slammer" in the restaurant industry. A slammer is known for the ability to turn out quality food at an accelerated pace.

But it is J.R.'s own struggle with food and weight that has endeared him to those who come to the Rice Diet Program. A self-described 400-pound kid, his weight eventually soared to nearly 700 pounds. J.R. first came to the program in '91 and lost significant weight. But like so many, he continued to fight the battle over the next years. He returned to Durham, lost weight, but eventually decided upon gastric-bypass surgery combined with the Rice Diet Program, which he credits with saving his life.

He's down to 270 pounds on his 6'2" frame and considers himself a work in progress. He took the job as Head Chef in '98. "I understand eating disorders and the fear and desperation that brings a patient to our doorway. In some small way, I think I can help. I can assure people that the fear which motivated them to come will pay off if they stick to the Program," says J.R. "I look at this as an opportunity for me to reassure and encourage patients at a time when it is so crucial. That's what I like best about the job."

Does he have a pet peeve? You bet. "I don't like it when patients lie to themselves and try to throw someone else off base. Sometimes they lose thirty pounds and become an expert. Let's face it. This is a lifetime commitment. People need to be realistic and follow the staff's advice. This program works. Guaranteed." J.R. notes that the program is salt and dairy free, but he does use herbs and seasonings to enhance flavor. His most requested recipes? Stuffed mushrooms, lasagna, garlic red skin potatoes, and his crab-free crabcakes. Take a peek in the recipe section!

# CHAPTER EIGHT

# CREATING OPTIMAL HEALTH

*Much of your pain is self chosen. It is the bitter potion by which the physician within you heals your sick self.*

—Kahlil Gibran

There's no doubt about it: The Rice Diet is the fastest and the surest way to better health and permanent weight loss. Whether you want to lose 20 pounds or 200, the Rice Diet will allow you to lose weight safely and gain health at the same time.

Most of the people who come to the Rice Diet Program come to lose weight. Once they are medically assessed, they often learn that they have been suffering from a host of other medical conditions such as heart disease and its precursors (hypertension, high cholesterol, diabetes, and abnormal sugar metabolism). They also suffer many of the other associated effects of obesity, such as sleep apnea, poor vision, and osteoarthritis. The Rice Diet can lessen, reverse, and even alleviate the symptoms of many of these conditions.

So while you may be most focused on your weight loss goals at the present time, we want you to see the amazing additional benefits that come from eating this way. You can lose weight on any diet that contains less calories than you have been eating to maintain, but this very low-saturated fat and low-sodium diet will inspire not only the fastest weight loss, but optimal health for the long run. In addition to summarizing some phenomenal results of our diets, we have also gathered the most current, relevant information regarding vitamins, minerals, and the use of antioxidants to improve health and prevent disease. You may be surprised at the healing power of the diet and at some of the recent findings!

# PREVENTING DISEASE

## CORONARY ARTERY DISEASE

The Rice Diet provides definitive treatment for coronary artery disease. It reverses every modifiable risk factor faster, safer and more effectively than any other proven treatment. It relieves the symptoms of coronary artery disease, angina pectoris, and congestive heart failure, and can make the use of drugs unnecessary. Indeed, we have witnessed numerous patients who arrive with congestive heart failure and reverse the symptoms of this disease in one to two weeks. As we've pointed out earlier, the beneficial effects of the diet on the risk factors that cause coronary artery disease—hypertension, high cholesterol, diabetes, and obesity—have been documented in Dr. Kempner's publications and confirmed by our own observations over the past twenty-two years. Other researchers have shown that lowering the cholesterol with diet or medication or both can lower the death rate from vascular disease. More recent studies have shown that lowering blood cholesterol can enhance regression of coronary artery blockages. And finally, in 1990, fifty-one years after Dr. Kempner began to use the Rice Diet clinically, Dr. Ornish and coworkers proved that coronary artery disease can be reversed with a low-fat diet similar to the Rice Diet.

The following case histories illustrate the power of the Rice Diet in treating patients with coronary artery disease and angina:

V.V., a fifty-five-year-old attorney, had undergone four-vessel coronary artery bypass surgery because of angina pectoris, but he developed recurrent angina, which persisted despite treatment with copious medications. Frustrated with his lack of progress, his doctors sent him to us.

When he arrived his blood pressure was elevated (165/98) even on medication, his fasting blood sugar was 194, his cholesterol 294, his triglycerides 183, and his heart size 15.2 centimeters. After one month on the diet, all of his blood measurements had decreased, showing rapid improvement: his blood pressure was 130/80 without medication, weight 157, fasting blood sugar 105, cholesterol 164 (down 130), and triglycerides 120. He had started on a walking program with no angina. Nine months later, his blood pressure was 137/81, his weight 140, and his heart size 11.1 centimeters (over one and one-half inches smaller). His medications were discontinued without an increase in his angina, and he was walking three to four hours a day without pain.

J.T. was fifty-nine years old when he came to the Rice Diet Program, having suffered from hypertension for fourteen years and angina for fifteen years. He had had a two-vessel aortocoronary bypass: but, his angina had recurred after five or six years. He had had another cardiac catheterization, which showed him to be inoperable. Even on medication, his angina persisted. At 222 pounds, he was in rough shape. And yet, after four weeks, he had lost 30 pounds, and both his blood sugar and cholesterol decreased. And although he stayed on some of his medications, he had no chest pain. After two months, we took him off his medications. He was walking two to three hours a day without pain!

# HYPERTENSION

The Rice Diet began as, and remains, an extremely effective treatment for high blood pressure. On the diet, patients can often completely stop medication use while maintaining the same or better control of their blood pressures. In a review of our recent patients, we found that we stopped all medication in 67 percent and decreased the amount or number of medications in an additional 19 percent. The average blood pressure fell from 149/89 to 134/79. So blood pressures can improve more dramatically on a no-salt vegetarian plus fish diet than on medications.

When Dr. Kempner first began using the diet, most of the patients he treated had what was called malignant hypertension. Blood pressures were commonly 220/150 or higher. Patients had symptoms caused by the blood pressure elevation such as headache, giddiness, shortness of breath, and chest pain. Severe changes were visible in the eyes (hemorrhages, exudates, and optic nerve swelling), changes on the electrocardiogram, and decreased kidney function. These patients usually died of stroke, heart attack, or kidney failure within three years. There were no effective medicines such as we have now. An operation called a bilateral lumbodorsal sympathectomy, in which all the sympathetic nerves to the legs were cut, was effective in about 10 percent of patients, but caused unpleasant and debilitating complications in many of the remainder.

Of the first five hundred patients treated with the Rice Diet, 60 to 75 percent improved. Moreover, the symptoms and signs associated with the elevated blood pressure sometimes improved before the blood pressure decreased appreciably suggesting that the brain, eye, heart, and kidney lesions were not caused by the elevated blood pressure alone. Also important, Dr. Kempner showed that it often took time for blood pressure to improve. Only 51 percent of his patients who were treated thirty-four days or less improved; whereas, 70 percent of those treated for longer periods improved.

As more patients were seen who have the kind of hypertension we see today, called essential hypertension, the success rate of the initial treatment rose to 82 percent: a success rate similar to that which we see today.

Though many medicines have become available for the treatment of hypertension, the medications themselves may cause problems. Many patients experience unpleasant side effects such as fatigue, weakness, and impotence. The medications have been shown to cause increases in cholesterol, blood sugar, and uric acid, and may even cause premature death.

Even if you are basically healthy, lower sodium intake can lower your blood pressure. This is important even if you have a "normal" blood pressure. On average, people with blood pressures of 90/60, versus so-called "normal" blood pressures of 120/80, have 30 percent less chance of having a cardiovascular event (heart attack or stroke). The lower your blood pressure the better (if you are not feeling dizzy upon standing), and the lower your sodium intake the lower your blood pressure. If your doctor says "you're normal," just remember that it is normal to die prematurely from a heart attack or a stroke in the industrialized world. Strive for your optimal, not "normal" in a very diseased population!

In four weeks, patients on the Rice Diet with normal blood pressures lowered their pressures from 118/75 to 113/71. Patients with undiagnosed hypertension (not on any meds) went from 149/90 to 122/74. This may not sound like much but a 5 to 20 point drop can be very significant in lowering your risk of heart attacks or strokes; researchers dream of such results. Plus, you will feel better when you eat less sodium. Most of us are carrying around 5 to 15 pounds of extra fluid. We are waterlogged. But we've gotten used to it, and only when we eat really high sodium food, such as Chinese food, can we appreciate how bad being waterlogged feels. When you cut back on sodium, the extra fluid leaves and you are no longer waterlogged and you feel better.

B.I. was forty-one when he came for treatment. His blood pressure was 140/100 and his weight was 218. In one month, his blood pressure was down to 120/80 and he had lost 30 pounds. In three months, his blood pressure was 105/80 and his weight was 143 (down 75 pounds).

F.B. was forty-nine years old when he came to the Rice Clinic with a five-year history of hypertension. His pressure was 181/112, despite being on two different medications. In sixteen days, he lost 14 pounds (256 to 242), all his medicines were stopped, and his blood pressure was 119/85!

# HIGH CHOLESTEROL

As mentioned earlier, elevated cholesterol is a major risk factor for heart and other vascular disease. The Rice Diet was the first effective treatment for high cholesterol. It lowered the cholesterol in 93 percent of patients with cholesterols above 220. Now we know that optimal cholesterol is below 200. It turns out that the diet lowers the cholesterol in over 90 percent of patients no matter what their cholesterol is to begin with.

It cannot be emphasized enough that saturated fat, not dietary cholesterol (which is the cholesterol that comes in food), is the most important factor in raising cholesterol. The serum cholesterol is affected by dietary cholesterol in only about one of every five people. Beware of products that advertise "no cholesterol"; many of these products are high in saturated fat and partially hydrogenated oils that are significantly more dangerous than dietary cholesterol itself. Even some monounsaturated oils can raise your cholesterol.

Reduce or eliminate saturated fats to lower your cholesterol: Saturated fat will raise blood cholesterol more predictably than any other substance, including dietary cholesterol. As you know, saturated fat is higher in animal products than in vegetables. The higher your saturated fat intake, the higher your blood cholesterol and the higher your risk of heart disease. If your cholesterol (or "bad cholesterol," called LDL-C) is high, less than 5 percent of your calories should come from saturated fats. Saturated fats have been shown to raise cholesterol about twice as much as mono- and polyunsaturated fats lower it.

Replace saturated fats with either healthy monounsaturated fats or omega-3 fats to improve cholesterol. Generally, when monounsaturated fats are used to replace saturated fats, blood cholesterol levels will decrease. But some monounsaturated fats seem to be more advantageous than others. Olive oil is highest in monounsaturated fats and has been shown to lower cholesterol as impressively as any other fat, without lowering the HDLs, as polyunsaturated fats tend to do. This is especially important for preventing heart disease in women, although more studies on women and heart disease need to be done. Since very low-fat diets, and polyunsaturated fat-rich diets not only lower cholesterol but also usually sacrifice significant amounts of HDLs, it might be to our benefit to enjoy a couple of teaspoons of olive oil daily, preferably uncooked. Canola oil appears to be the lowest in saturated fat, though it has not been proven to lower cholesterol without lowering HDLs, as much as has olive oil. But not all monounsaturated fats can be recommended. Peanut oil is one worthy of note. Although peanut oil does not appear to be that high in saturated fat, it has been shown to raise cholesterol and produce atherosclerosis in animal studies. So for those wanting spreadable nut butter, try using small amounts of tahini, ground sesame seeds (usually sold in ethnic sections of chain grocery stores), or almond butter (found in health food stores). When polyunsaturated fats are used in place of saturated fats, blood cholesterol decreases. This is not to suggest that large amounts would be recommended, since all fats contain some saturated fatty acids, and polyunsaturated fats have been shown to lower HDLs as well as LDLs. In fact, large amounts of polyunsaturated fats are thought to increase the risk of free-radical damage, which has been connected with cancer, heart disease, and many immune system functions. Walnuts, almonds, and sesame seeds are a few examples of polyunsaturated fats that can be enjoyed in moderation.

There can be no doubt now that lowering cholesterol in humans causes regression of atherosclerosis (blockages in arteries). Although the cholesterol usually decreases most markedly in the first month of treatment, it may take quite some time as with hypertension. The reduction in cholesterol usually becomes greater with time. One patient, S.H., came to us with a cholesterol of 400 and a triglyceride of 2336. (Triglycerides are the way we carry fats in our blood and store them in our fat cells. They are elevated as part of the now much discussed metabolic syndrome.) His weight was 221. After one week on the Basic Rice Diet, he had lost 9 pounds, his cholesterol was 290, and his triglyceride 790. He went home on a modified diet and returned nineteen days later for a checkup with a weight of 201, a cholesterol of 158, and a triglyceride of 288!

# DIABETES

The Rice Diet has helped countless patients with diabetes. In many, clinical symptoms of diabetes entirely disappear; in others, insulin requirements fall and the complications of diabetes are lessened or eliminated.

There are two primary types of diabetes. Type 1 diabetes, which does not usually run in the family, begins early in life (usually by age twenty), may occur in thin or overweight patients, and requires insulin to prevent death. All these patients are really insulin dependent. Type 2 diabetes usually runs in the family, begins later in life, is associated with being overweight, and can be controlled by diet and exercise or pills; although many patients who do not lose weight and increase their exercise eventually require insulin to control their blood sugars.

The main problems in diabetes are the complications caused by an uncontrolled elevated blood sugar over time. Diabetics may develop bleeding in their eyes (diabetic retinopathy). In fact, diabetes is the leading cause of blindness in adults. Diabetics have an acceleration of vascular disease so that they are more likely to have strokes, angina pectoris, heart attacks, and intermittent claudication (pain in the legs with exercise caused by blockages in the arteries to the legs). Diabetes can cause kidney disease (diabetic nephropathy) and is the leading reason why patients need dialysis or kidney transplant. Diabetics can have trouble with their nerves (diabetic neuropathy), which causes pain, difficulty feeling, double vision, stomach and bowel problems, and impotence. They often have trouble fighting infection and healing. The tragedies of diabetic complications are dramatically compounded when you realize how most of them could have been prevented.

*Note:* If you have diabetes—since diabetics have a two-to three-fold higher risk for heart disease than nondiabetics, they should be especially mindful of increasing their soluble fiber intake. Soluble fiber—rich foods will not only improve their diabetes management by reducing insulin requirements, increasing insulin sensitivity, and stabilizing blood sugars, but will significantly reduce other risk factors for disease such as high cholesterol, LDLs, triglycerides, and obesity.

Control of the blood sugar is the key to preventing these complications. The Rice Diet helps to treat and prevent all of the complications of diabetes and of the other risk factors (i.e., high blood pressure) that augment the damage caused by the elevated blood sugar.

The success of the Rice Diet in patients with diabetes has been well documented in medical literature. A number of patients came to Dr. Kempner because they were blinded by diabetic retinopathy. N.C. was such a patient. She was twenty-five years old when she first came to Dr. Kempner in 1983. She had had diabetes since she was nine years old. I remember her telling me that when she sat next to Dr. Kempner she could not see his face. Six months later, she had a day-driver's license!

K.Q. was forty-eight years old when he came to the Rice Diet Program because of diabetes and diabetic neuropathy. He had developed leg pain about two years prior to coming. Because of both high blood sugar and high blood pressure, he was taking medications. At the time of his arrival, he weighed 254 pounds, his blood pressure was 126/76, and his blood sugars before breakfast, lunch, and supper were 200, 265, and 241, respectively. Most diabetics use a glucometer to check their own blood sugars one or more times a day.

As soon as he started the Rice Diet, his medications were stopped. One month later, his weight was 225, blood pressure 130/84, and cholesterol 144. He continued on the diet, though he came only intermittently to see us. After six months, his weight was 182, blood pressure 112/76, blood sugars before breakfast, lunch, and dinner 90, 84, and 78, respectively, and cholesterol 149. His leg pain was 90 percent improved.

Until the end of the 1970s, it was believed that except for sugar (sucrose), all carbohydrates had the same effect on the blood sugar. But, in recent years, the blood sugar response to various foods has been examined more closely. It has been shown that unlike carbohydrate-rich foods that rapidly elevate the blood sugar and stimulate insulin secretion, certain soluble fiber-rich, high-carbohydrate foods are slowly absorbed and actually stabilize blood sugars and reduce insulin responses.

Thus, dietary recommendations for diabetes now recommend "a diet high in complex carbohydrate and soluble fiber, and low in fat." The Rice Diet, which is rich in fiber, fits the bill. Research shows that whole foods produce a diminished and more gradual rise in blood glucose than do their more refined counterparts. For instance, cracked wheat or bulgur is more slowly absorbed than whole wheat bread, and whole wheat bread is more slowly absorbed than white

## THE FRINGE BENEFITS

Though we have concrete evidence to support how the Rice Diet improves diabetes, kidney disease, heart disease and its risk factors, including obesity, we have also noticed a number of other health improvements over the years. We can't say for sure that it's the Rice Diet behind the cure, but it sure seems that way!

Take a look at these conditions that disappeared or lessened when on the Rice Diet:

· It is now recognized that many people who are overweight develop liver disease. The initial stage is fatty infiltration of the liver, which then progresses to a kind of hepatitis (non-alcoholic steatohepatitis or NASH), and eventually to cirrhosis of the liver. The weight loss and exercise regimen of the Rice Diet certainly helps this problem.

• Polycystic Ovary disease is associated with high insulin levels. As you lose weight on the Rice Diet, you will most likely see an improvement in your condition.

• Since celiac is gluten induced, and we don't serve gluten here (with the exception of pasta and shredded wheat, which you can simply not eat), this is a good choice of diets for those with celiac disease.

• We have had lots of experience treating patients with fibromyalgia. By taking better care of yourself (eating right, sensible exercise), you can get better. Our experience has been very positive.

• Because the Rice Diet is a high-fiber diet, it can help manage irritable bowel syndrome (IBS). Also, one of the symptoms of IBS is loose stools, and the rice, oatmeal, and fruit are common choices here that usually slow bowel movements.

In addition, we have seen improvements with such conditions as sleep apnea, psoriasis, pulmonary hypertension, edema, and stiffness in the joints associated with arthritis. On the Rice Diet you will lose weight, probably more than you imagined possible. But you will also get healthier eating this way. For anyone interested in discovering more about the health benefits of the Rice Diet Program, especially anyone concerned about heart disease and its precursors, take a look at Kitty's book, *Heal Your Heart* (Wiley, 1997).

bread. One study that examined the blood sugar response to identical portions of beans processed by different methods found the blood sugars were 50 percent lower in the beans with unruptured cells when compared to those beans with ruptured cells. More evidence that we benefit from consuming whole foods rather than their processed products.

# WAYS TO IMPROVE YOUR OVERALL HEALTH

The Rice Diet will undoubtedly improve your overall health and help prevent, reverse, or mitigate all of the health conditions described above. The following is a summary of other specific ways to improve your health and reduce your concerns with weight, diabetes, cancer, cholesterol, osteoporosis, and free-radical damage (associated with cancer, heart disease, and other health risks):

• **Limit your sodium intake:** Sodium intakes averaging from 500 to 1,000 milligrams per day prevent many health problems besides the commonly known ones: high blood pressure, kidney disease, and congestive heart failure. In a review of studies on salt and carbohydrate metabolism, Egan and Lackland (2000) note that cross-cultural studies of people with low-sodium intakes show a low occurrence of high blood pressure, as well as disorders of fat and carbohydrate metabolism. There is significant scientific evidence that shows that if you eat something with salt you have a higher blood glucose rise and plasma insulin response, thus absorb more calories from it, than if you eat it without added salt. This was demonstrated by Dr. Anne Thorburn and associates in research that showed increasing sodium intake significantly increased the glucose and insulin response after a meal. This study suggests that adding salt to your food could only make matters worse for diabetics and overweight people trying to lose weight.

• **Increase your fiber:** Increasing our fiber intake has been linked to the reduction of many prevalent diseases including hiatal hernia, hemorrhoids, diverticular disease, irritable bowel syndrome, constipation, gallbladder disease, and heart disease (and many of its risk factors such as obesity, diabetes, high cholesterol, high blood pressure, and high triglycerides). On the Rice Diet, triglycerides do increase in about 15 percent of patients, but they decrease with longer times on the diet and with further weight loss.

• **Increase omega-3s:** Omega-3 fatty acids are a type of polyunsaturated fat thought to be beneficial for preventing heart disease and its risk factors, as well as cancer, autoimmune diseases, and inflammatory diseases such as arthritis. Some studies show omega-3 fatty acids lower cholesterol, but most of them show more significant reductions in blood pressure and triglycerides. Omega-3 fatty acids also help prevent blood clots and coronary artery spasms, which are two underlying causes of heart attacks. High amounts of omega-3 fatty acids are found in oilier fish (such as mackerel, salmon, trout, bluefish, and tuna).

• **Improve your bone density:** Although consuming inadequate calcium is a risk factor for osteoporosis, so are many other factors that may have more importance than our calcium intake, especially when you consider their accumulative effect. The dairy industry has plenty of money to sell you on how cool it is to have milk on your upper lip. But the companies or farms that would benefit from your knowing these other risk factors of osteoporosis don't have the resources to educate us through commercial advertising or to afford lobbyists for governmental policy decisions that are truly based on health facts. But, to make a long story short, the other risk factors of osteoporosis that are important are:

- Consuming excessive sodium, animal protein, phosphates (from soda and meat), caffeine and alcohol intake.

- Inadequate weight-bearing and muscle-strengthening exercises.

- Smoking cigarettes.

Few people know that high sodium, sodas, and meat (phosphate) intake greatly increase our risk of developing osteoporosis (because Mrs. Dash and the many fledgling no-sodium condiment companies, the bean and pea industry, and herbal teas don't have the money to educate us on their healthier products). A further development in this area is the research on the implications of the ratio of animal to plant sources of protein on bone health. A seven-year follow-up study of 1,035 women over age sixty-five showed that a high ratio of animal to vegetable protein in the diet was associated with more rapid deterioration of the femoral neck bone and a greater risk of hip fracture. These results suggest that an increase in vegetable protein sources, such as beans and peas, and reduction in animal sources may decrease bone loss and risk of hip fracture.

Despite the fact that Americans have been led to believe that dairy is going to save them from osteoporosis, the international data does not support this hypothesis. Although dairy products are an excellent source of calcium, their high protein and sodium content depletes significant amounts, making vegetarian sources of calcium all the more attractive. Calcium is found in high amounts in healthier foods, such as greens (especially collards, kale, turnip greens, and spinach), dried beans (especially black turtle beans, and tofu or soymilk with added calcium), broccoli, rhubarb, blackstrap molasses, and amaranth.

If you have a bone density suggesting osteoporosis or osteopenia, or a family history of either, it would be to your advantage to supplement with calcium unless you want to ensure dairy, fortified soy products, and the above rich sources at every meal. While possible to obtain calcium from natural sources, those with osteoporosis or osteopenia will likely find weight loss easier if they supplement, or else eat mega-servings of dark green leafy vegetables. Obviously, the more natural calcium-rich food sources, exercise (aerobic and muscle strengthening), and stress management practice, the better for preventing osteoporosis; as with other diseases, it is wiser and easier to prevent than to reverse. Although there are nutritional and health benefits of nonfat yogurt, the advantages of soy milk over cow's milk are significant. While containing similar amounts of protein and calcium (some fortified varieties of soy milk contain even more), soy milk contains significantly more thiamin, niacin, magnesium, copper, and manganese. Furthermore, you don't have to wonder about how many antibiotics and hormones the cow was dosed with. Eating "lower on the food chain" inspires more health for you, others, and the planet. Just open your mind and try West Soy Plus on your next cereal. My son was weaned on it and refuses to drink cow's milk—and he has not been informed of the above information!

## WHICH FOODS ARE RICH IN ANTIOXIDANTS?

Antioxidants are abundant in fruits and vegetables, as well as in other foods including nuts, grains, and some meats, poultry, and fish. The list below describes food sources of common antioxidants.

• **Beta-carotene** is found in many foods that are orange in color, including sweet potatoes, carrots, cantaloupe, squash, apricots, pumpkin, and mangoes. Most green, leafy vegetables including collard greens, spinach, and kale are also rich in beta-carotene.

• **Lutein,** best known for its association with healthy eyes, is abundant in green, leafy vegetables such as collard greens, spinach, and kale.

• **Lycopene** is a potent antioxidant found in tomatoes, watermelon, guava, papaya, apricots, pink grapefruit, blood oranges, and other foods. Estimates suggest 85 percent of American dietary intake of lycopene comes from tomatoes and tomato products.

• **Selenium** is a mineral and a component of antioxidant enzymes. Plant foods like rice and wheat are the major dietary sources of selenium in most countries. The amount of selenium in soil, which varies by region, determines the amount of selenium in the foods grown in that soil. Animals that eat grains or plants grown in selenium-rich soil have higher levels of selenium in their muscle. In the United States, meats and bread are common sources of dietary selenium. Brazil nuts also contain large quantities of selenium.

• **Vitamin C** is also called ascorbic acid, and can be found in abundance in most fruits and vegetables, especially citrus fruits.

• **Vitamin E,** also known as alpha-tocopherol, is found in olive oil, almonds (and many other nuts and seeds), wheat germ, and soybean products.

• **Take your vitamins and minerals** to ensure optimal functioning of your body and cells. Vitamins and minerals are micronutrients that may benefit your body needs for normal growth, function, and health. Vitamins help in growth, digestion, mental alertness, and resistance to infection. They also enable our bodies to use the macronutrients we are eating—the carbohydrates, fats, and proteins—and act as catalysts for metabolism. Minerals are the main components in your teeth and bones. They help in the generation of cells and enzymes; regulate the balance of body fluids; control the movement of nerve impulses; and deliver oxygen to cells and take away carbon dioxide. We get all the vitamins and minerals from the foods we eat on the Rice Diet, if our daily choices include milk (soy enriched with calcium), beans, and dark green leafy vegetables. However, we recommend that you take a multivitamin supplement to boost your intake and insure your daily requirements for health are being met. It serves as an insurance policy since many of us are not eating exclusively organic, locally grown, fresh fruits and vegetables; the nutritional quality of our produce is questionable otherwise.

• **Fight free radicals with foods rich in antioxidants** such as beta-carotene, lutein, lycopene, selenium, and vitamins E and C. Every day millions of free radicals are formed in the body. Normal essential bodily processes often initiate them, but environmental forces such as cigarette smoke, car exhaust, and ultraviolet light might also initiate them. Antioxidants have been associated with a reduction in free-radical damage that has been implicated in cancerous growths, undesirable skin changes such as wrinkling, cataracts, arthritis, neuromuscular disorders, and in the oxidation of LDL (which is a major factor in the atherosclerosis process). The free-radical theory is not a new one, but the growing volume of research on the dangers of free radicals and our defenses against them is both inspiring and newsworthy. The theory was originally proposed in 1956 and states that free radicals produced by cellular metabolism cause the progressive accumulation of degenerative changes that over a period of time are responsible for the undesirable processes that accompany aging. It's best to get your antioxidants from the whole foods themselves because of both their other health benefits and because research is showing mixed results of taking antioxidants in supplement form. The following tips summarize how to reduce our oxidized fats and increase our antioxidant intake:

- Limit saturated fat intake (from meats, sauces, dressings, desserts), and use the monounsaturated fatty acid–rich oils such as olive and canola oils.

- Avoid fried foods, especially in restaurants where the oil in the fat fryers can go unchanged for weeks. Fat that has been heated to high temperature is very volatile and saturated with oxygen. Oxidized fats contribute to atherosclerosis, the underlying cause of most heart disease.

- Make a point of eating fresh fruits and vegetables, preferably at least three fruits and six vegetables every day. The root and dark green, leafy vegetables are especially high in vitamins E, C, and beta-carotene.

The National Cancer Institute recently reported on five large-scale clinical trials published in the 1990s that reached differing conclusions on the effect of antioxidants on cancer. The research on the supplementation of antioxidants shows that they don't consistently help and can even hinder your health, which is why we recommend you get your antioxidants from the foods you eat. In a meta-analysis of seven studies for the prevention of gastrointestinal cancers, 131,727 people were randomized into either antioxidant vitamin treatment group or a placebo (control) group. In comparison to the placebo group, there was a significantly higher death rate in the vitamin group. The results are also inconsistent in the recent research on heart disease performed by the Heart Protection Study. The more research we read, the more incredibly naïve it seems to assume we know enough about what we need from food to believe we can encapsulate it without risks. Even when we have large, well-designed studies, the results and opinions tend to vary, but seem to come back to the recommendation to primarily trust what grows (organically) from the ground and swims in the water.

# INSPIRATIONAL CORNER: A FOUR-GENERATION RICE DIET FAMILY

Mr. and Mrs. H., both suffering from cardiovascular disease, had been on the Rice Diet for four months. Their son N., with his wife, F., and two children, came to Durham in 1956 to visit them for Christmas. The son arrived with a heavy heart, knowing that his doctors at home had virtually given up on his sixty-year-old father, who had hypertension, kidney disease, and heart failure. When N. and his family arrived at the hotel to meet his parents, they were stunned by the trim, energetic man who strode grinning across the lobby to greet them. "It was Pop!" N. exclaims. "It knocked me to my knees."

Contrary to all expectations, with the Rice Diet reversals of his diseases, Mr. H. lived another ten active years, traveling the world and wintering in Florida.

During that visit, N.'s parents urged him to try out the diet, too, just while he was in town. At thirty-seven, he already had hypertension, which was gradually worsening despite medication; genes from both parents predisposed him to vascular disease. Reluctantly, N. submitted to a physical and he and his wife spent the next ten days eating rice and fruit. N.'s blood pressure went from 157/91 (with anti-hypertensive drugs) to 107/74 (without drugs). He was impressed, but still dubious: As a busy executive who conducted much of his business over lunch, he couldn't imagine maintaining "this cockamamey regime" at home. But he gave it a good disciplined effort and returned to the Rice House six months later a confirmed believer, 20 pounds lighter, with good blood pressure, and a smaller heart. The couple found that incorporating the diet into their life was not as big a challenge as they'd feared. In fact, N.'s business associates often followed his example in ordering healthy salads and fruit plates for lunch.

Forty-eight years later, N. and F. came back to Durham for their annual visit to the Rice House. At eighty-five, N. is as slim as a teenager and full of energy. His wife, F., petite and lovely, has been slowed a little—temporarily, we hope—by a couple of bad falls. They described how they themselves have not only been faithful followers of the Rice Diet regime but have passed it down as a way of life to their children, raising their son and daughter on a low-fat, sodium-free diet (with some flexibility away from home). Their daughter, a lawyer, "still lunches at her desk with a box of Shredded Wheat," says N., and has raised her own family on a low-sodium, low-fat diet. And, added F., their son, now sixty, was on his way to join them for a few days to get his own Rice Diet tune-up.

N. retired twenty-two years ago from his second successful business enterprise, but he hasn't appreciably slowed down: he's been head of his local chapter of the Service Corps of Retired Executives, president of his homeowners' association, and, with F., a tireless traveler. In the last two years alone, they've visited Papua New Guinea, Afghanistan, Iran, Cambodia, and Laos; they've followed the Silk Route and climbed ruins in Central America. Not bad for someone who, nearly half a century ago, already felt threatened by heart disease.

# CHAPTER NINE

# THE RECIPES AND WEEKLY MENUS

*Let me tell you the secret that has led to my goal. My strength lies solely in my tenacity.*

—LOUIS PASTEUR

The Rice Diet Program is fortunate to have a long history of delicious, inspired meals. The following recipes offer a compilation of some of the favorite Rice House Recipes, many by Chef J.R. and Nancy, as well as those created by Dr. Rosati himself, which, of course, tend to be inspired by his Italian heritage. A few of these are compliments of other friends and me (Kitty).

Other wonderful additions to our Rice Diet Program recipes come from our valued dietitian, Rachelle Fong, MS, MPH, RD, LDN. Rachelle teaches nutrition classes, provides participants with nutritional counseling, and helps them develop a plan for going home. She also offers interactive, energetic cooking classes in which Rice Diet participants learn how to prepare foods that are tasty and healthy. The recipes that follow are those that Rachelle has long made for her family and friends, molded now to fit within the Rice Diet guidelines. Being raised as a third-generation Asian American in California, Rachelle's recipes have an Asian flair and a special attention to presentation. All the recipes are followed by a nutritional analysis; note all seafood recipes include their omega-3 fatty acid content.

Enjoy!

# WEEKLY MENUS

Here are a week's worth of menus for each of the three phases of the Rice Diet. All recipes printed in italic are included in the following chapters.

# RICE DIET PHASE ONE WEEKLY MENU

| Meals | Sunday | Monday | Tuesday |
|---|---|---|---|
| | 1,000 Calories | 800 Calories | 1,000 Calories |
| **Breakfast** | Ezekiel 4:9 bread, 1 slice<br><br>1 cup nonfat yogurt<br><br>Bionature Fruite Spread, 2 tablespoons | Irish (steel-cut) oats, 1 cup<br><br>Raisins, 2 tablespoons<br><br>Pineapple, 1 cup | Granola, ⅓ cup<br><br>1 cup nonfat yogurt<br><br>Berries, 1 cup |
| **Lunch** | *Black Bean and Corn Salad*<br><br>Tomato, sliced, 1 cup<br><br>*Balsamic Dressing*<br><br>Melba toast, 2<br><br>*Grilled Peach* | Brown basmati rice, ⅔ cup<br><br>Fresh fruit salad, 1 cup<br><br>1 peach | *Black Beans and Corn Salad*<br><br>Salad, 2 cups<br><br>Melba toast, 2<br><br>*Balsamic Dressing*<br><br>Pear, 1 |
| **Dinner** | *Wild Rice Salad*<br><br>Lettuce Salad Bed, 2½ cups<br><br>Chick peas, ⅓ cup<br><br>*Balsamic Dressing*<br><br>Fresh fruit salad, 1 cup | Brown basmati rice, ⅔ cup<br><br>Melon, 1 cup<br><br>Berries, 1 cup | Inca red quinoa, 1 cup<br><br>Stir Fry Vegetables, 1½ cups<br><br>Mr. Spice Ginger Stir Fry Sauce, 2 tablespoons<br><br>Fruit salad, 1 cup |

| Wednesday | Thursday | Friday | Saturday |
|---|---|---|---|
| 1,000 Calories | 1,000 Calories | 1,000 Calories | 1,000 Calories |
| Cereal, ¾ cup<br><br>Soy milk, 1 cup<br><br>Banana, ½ | Cereal, ¾ cup<br><br>Skim milk, 1 cup<br><br>Banana, ½ | Cereal, ¾ cup<br><br>Soy milk, 1 cup<br><br>Dried cherries,<br>2 tablespoons | Ezekiel 4:9 bread,<br>1 slice<br><br>Bionaturae Organic<br>Plum Spread,<br>2 tablespoons<br><br>Soy milk, 1 cup |
| Health Valley<br>Vegetarian Chili,<br>1 cup<br><br>Lime juice and<br>cilantro<br><br>Salad, 2 cups<br><br>*Balsamic Dressing*<br><br>Fruit salad, 1 cup | Chinese restaurant<br>order:<br><br>Steamed rice,<br>1 cup<br><br>Stir-fried vegetables<br>(sauteed with sake,<br>extra garlic, ginger;<br>no fat, soy sauce, or<br>MSG), 1½ cups<br><br>Fresh fruit, 1 piece | Baked potato,<br>1 medium<br><br>Vegetable salad,<br>3 cups<br><br>*Balsamic Dressing*,<br>2 tablespoons<br><br>Melon, 1 cup | Quinoa pasta,<br>1 cup<br><br>Marco Polo Sauce,<br>⅔ cup<br><br>Tossed salad,<br>3 cups<br><br>Consorzio Raspberry<br>Balsamic Dressing,<br>2 tablespoons<br><br>Fruit salad, 1 cup |
| Black Pearl Medley,<br>1 cup<br><br>Desert Pepper<br>Peach Mango Salsa,<br>4 tablespoons<br><br>Tossed salad,<br>2 cups<br><br>Berries, ½ cup | Fusilli, 1½ cups<br><br>Spaghetti sauce,<br>low-sodium, 1 cup<br><br>Salad, 1½ cups<br><br>Consorzio Raspberry<br>Balsamic Dressing<br><br>Melon, 1 cup | Corn or flour tortilla<br><br>Bearitos, refried<br><br>Beans with lime and<br>cilantro and chilis<br>½ cup<br><br>Enrico's Chunky<br>Salsa, 5 tablespoons<br><br>Salad, 2 cups<br><br>*Grilled Peach* | *Rachelle's Mexican<br>Baked Beans*<br><br>Rice, ⅓ cup<br><br>*Spinach Salad with<br>Oranges*, 2 cups<br><br>*Balsamic Dressing*,<br>1 tablespoon |

# RICE DIET PHASE TWO WEEKLY MENU

| Meals | Sunday | Monday, basic rice | Tuesday |
|---|---|---|---|
| | 1,000 Calories | 800 Calories | 1,000 Calories |
| **Breakfast** | Blueberry Banana Muffin<br><br>1 cup yogurt | Oatmeal, 1 cup<br><br>Dried cherries,<br>1 tablespoon<br><br>Melon, 1 cup | ¾ cup cereal<br><br>1 cup skim milk<br><br>Raisins,<br>1 tablespoon<br><br>Strawberries, ½ cup |
| **Lunch** | Black Beans and Garlic<br><br>Basmati rice,<br>⅓ cup<br><br>Taco Salad<br><br>Bok Choy | Brown rice, ⅔ cup<br><br>Mixed berries,<br>1½ cup | Basmati rice,<br>½ cup<br><br>Black Beans and Garlic<br><br>Baked Eggplant Slices<br><br>Tomato Sauce,<br>½ cup<br><br>Blueberries, ¾ cup |
| **Dinner** | Baked Eggplant Slices<br><br>Swiss Chard<br><br>Southwest Corn<br><br>Fruit salad, 1 cup | Blueberry-Banana Muffin<br><br>Basmati rice,<br>⅔ cup<br><br>Fresh fruit, 1 piece | JR's Lasagna<br><br>Baby Greens with Roasted Bell Peppers<br><br>Melon, ½ cup |

| Wednesday | Thursday | Friday | Saturday, veg. plus |
|---|---|---|---|
| 1,000 Calories | 1,000 Calories | 1,000 Calories | 1,200 Calories |
| Blueberry-Banana Muffin<br><br>1 cup nonfat yogurt<br><br>Melon, ¾ cup | Cereal, ¾ cup<br><br>1 cup skim milk<br><br>Berries, ½ cup<br><br>Raisins, 1 tablespoon | Blueberry Peach Cobbler<br><br>¾ cup yogurt<br><br>Strawberries, ⅔ cup | Cereal, ¾ cup<br><br>1 cup skim milk<br><br>Strawberries ½ cup<br><br>Dried Cherries, 1 tablespoon |
| JR's Lasagna<br><br>Spinach Salad/ Mandarin Orange<br><br>Balsamic Dressing, 2 tablespoons<br><br>Garlic Roasted Veggies<br><br>Berries, ¾ cup | Rachelle's Barley and Lentil Salad<br><br>Swiss Chard<br><br>Matzo cracker<br><br>Melon, 1 cup | Rice House Meatloaf<br><br>Broccoli Rabe<br><br>Berries, 1 cup | Asparagus-Spinach Salad<br><br>Rachelle's Curried Lentil Soup with Mango<br><br>Basmati rice, ⅔ cup<br><br>Fresh fruit salad, ¾ cup |
| Split Pea Soup<br><br>Black Pearl medley, 1 cup<br><br>Broccoli Rabe<br><br>Fruit Salad, ½ cup | Split Pea Soup<br><br>Stuffed Artichokes<br><br>Garlic Red Skin Potatoes<br><br>Fresh fruit, 1 piece | Rachelle's Curried Lentil Soup with Mango<br><br>Creamed Spinach<br><br>Sweet Potato Pie, ½ serving | Crispy Flounder<br><br>Garlic Red Skin Potatoes<br><br>Shitake Slaw<br><br>Creamed Spinach<br><br>Grilled Peach |

# RICE DIET PHASE THREE WEEKLY MENU

| Meals | Sunday | Monday | Tuesday |
|-------|--------|--------|---------|
|  | 1,200 Calories | 800 Calories | 1,000 Calories |
| **Breakfast** | Irish (steel-cut) oatmeal, 1 cup<br><br>Raisins, 1 tablespoon<br><br>Berries, 1 cup | Irish (steel-cut) oatmeal, 1 cup<br><br>Fresh fruit salad, 1 cup<br><br>Dried cherries, 2 tablespoons | Cereal, ¾ cup<br><br>Nonfat soy or grain milk, 1 cup<br><br>Berries, 1 cup |
| **Lunch** | *Italian Bread Salad*<br><br>*Bruschetta with White Beans*<br><br>Mixed baby greens, 1 cup<br><br>*Roasted Peppers*<br><br>Grapes, 12 frozen | Brown basmati rice, ⅔ cup<br><br>Pineapple chunks, 1 cup<br><br>Banana, ½ piece | Baked Potato, small<br><br>Tossed Salad, 3 cups of veggies: bell peppers, carrots, tomatoes, and vinegar<br><br>Chickpeas, ⅓ cup<br><br>Fresh fruit, 1 piece |
| **Dinner** | *Vegetarian Ragu*<br><br>*Chess' Roasted Artichoke Salad*<br><br>*Clementines and Strawberries with Vinegar and Pepper* | Brown basmati rice, ⅔ cup<br><br>Mixed berries, 1 cup<br><br>Melon, 1 cup | *Sprout Packed Spring Rolls,* 4 pieces<br><br>*Clementines and Strawberries with Vinegar and Pepper* |

| Wednesday | Thursday | Friday | Saturday |
|---|---|---|---|
| 1000 Calories | 1,000 Calories | 1,000 Calories | 1,200 Calories |
| Cereal, ¾ cup<br><br>Skim milk, 1 cup<br><br>Raisins,<br>1 tablespoon<br><br>Blueberries, ½ cup | Granola, ⅓ cup<br><br>Puffed Wheat, ½ cup<br><br>Skim milk, 1 cup<br><br>Berries, ½ cup | Ezekiel 4:9 bread,<br>1 slice<br><br>Dry curd cottage<br>cheese, ½ cup<br><br>Bionature Plum<br>Spread,<br>1 tablespoon | Puffed Wheat, 1 cup<br><br>Nature's Path Hemp<br>Plus Granola,<br>⅓ cup<br><br>Apple juice, ½ cup |
| *Sprout Packed*<br>*Spring Rolls,*<br>4 pieces<br><br>*Kitty's Low Sodium*<br>*Soy Sauce Dip,*<br>2 tablespoons<br><br>Melon, 1 cup | Chinese<br>restaurant order:<br><br>Steamed rice, 1 cup<br><br>Stir-fried vegetables<br>in sake with extra<br>garlic, ginger, and<br>no soy sauce or<br>MSG, 1½ cups<br><br>Apple, 1 medium | *Chestnut Cornbread*<br>*Cranberry Stuffing*<br><br>Tossed Salad, 1 cup<br><br>*Balsamic Dressing*<br><br>Fresh fruit salad, 1<br>cup | *Lentil Quinoa Salad*<br><br>Vegetable Salad,<br>1½ cups<br><br>*Balsamic Dressing*<br><br>Pear, 1 piece |
| *Chestnut Cornbread*<br>*Cranberry Stuffing*<br><br>*Baby Greens and*<br>*Roasted Peppers*<br><br>Fresh fruit salad,<br>½ cup | Corn or flour tortilla<br><br>Bearitos, refried<br>beans, ⅔ cup<br><br>Enrico's No-Salt<br>Salsa, ½ cup<br><br>Tossed salad, 2 cups<br><br>*Balsamic Dressing*<br><br>Pear, 1 piece | *Marinated Tofu*<br>*Cutlets,* 2 slices or<br>3 ounces tofu<br><br>Brown basmati rice,<br>½ cup<br><br>Asparagus spears,<br>8 pieces<br><br>*Grilled Peaches* | *Mackerel Brushetta*<br><br>*Swordfish Risotto*<br><br>*Broccoli with Garlic*<br>*and White Wine*<br><br>*Grilled Peaches* |

# BASICS

The following recipes can help you create tasty dishes to combine with others or enjoy on their own.

## ARUGULA PESTO (WITH PASTA)

As an alternative to basil, use arugula for a flavorful—and nutritious—pesto for pasta (recipe below), polenta, or gnocchi. You can also make this pesto with spinach!

2 cups arugula leaves, cleaned (or spinach/basil)
1 cup parsley, freshly chopped
2 tablespoons toasted pine nuts
2 teaspoons grated pecorino cheese
2 teaspoons grated parmesan cheese
4 garlic cloves, roughly chopped
1 tablespoon extra virgin olive oil
Pepper to taste
1 pound pasta

Combine the ingredients, except for the pasta, in a food processor until a paste is formed. Boil pasta; any type is fine, but the more crevices the pasta has for the pesto to adhere to the better!

YIELD: 8 servings

**Each serving contains approximately:** Calories 240, Fat calories 33, Fat 3.7 g, Saturated fat 0.7 g, Cholesterol 1 mg, Protein 9 g, Carbohydrate 44 g, Dietary fiber 2 g, Sodium 24 mg, Calories from fat 14%, Calories from saturated fat 3%

**Allowances:** ⅝ fat + 2⅕ starches + ⅕ vegetable

**Those with heart disease reversal goals should omit cheese and substitute walnuts for pine nuts. Without cheese, each serving contains approximately**: Calories 235, Fat calories 31, Total fat 3.4 g, Saturated fat 0.6 g, Cholesterol 0 mg, Protein 8 g, Carbohydrate 44 g, Dietary fiber 2 g, Sodium 9 mg, Calories from fat 13%, Calories from saturated fat 2%

# TUSCAN BREAD

You may not remember the last time you tasted homemade bread, but when you try this recipe, you will never forget! This bread has a wonderful tasty crust and a delectable center. You can use it for bruschetta or toast in the morning.

2 packages fast-rising dry yeast
2½ cups tepid water (about 110 degrees)
6½ cups unbleached white-bread flour (do not use all-purpose flour)
⅛ cup cornmeal or semolina flour (to flour the board)

Dissolve the yeast in the water and let stand 5 minutes. Add 4 cups of the flour to make a batter, stirring to help it dissolve. Beat for 10 minutes with the paddle of an electric mixer or until the batter pulls away from the sides of the mixing bowl, or mix by hand if you prefer. Add the remaining flour and knead for 5 minutes in a machine using a dough hook, or approximately 15 minutes by hand. The cornmeal or semolina flour can be used as needed to dust your kneading surface. You may need to add more water to get a moist, elastic dough.

Leave the dough on a piece of plastic wrap, and cover with a large metal bowl. Allow the dough to rise until doubled, which will take 1 to 2 hours. Punch down the dough with your fists, folding it over a few times into a nice mound, and let rise for another 1½ hours.

Punch down again, then cut dough into three sections, molding them into loaves. Place the loaves on a floured cotton towel, dust them with a little more flour, then cover with another floured cotton towel. Preheat the oven to 450 degrees and place a pan of hot water on the bottom oven shelf. When the loaves have doubled in volume again, place them in the upper third of the oven, upside down, where the bottom is now the top and vice versa. Bake for approximately 25 minutes or until the crust is slightly browned and the loaves sound hollow when thumped. Cool on a rack before slicing.

YIELD: 40 slices

**Each serving contains approximately:** Calories 84, Fat calories 3, Fat .25 g, Saturated fat 0 g, Cholesterol 0 g, Protein 3 g, Carbohydrate 17 g, Dietary fiber 1 g, Sodium 1 mg, Calories of fat 3%, Calories from saturated fat 0%

**Allowances:** 1 starch

# KITTY'S CORNBREAD

Joy Nelson of Tyler, Texas, was an angel in helping us with heart-healthy recipes, and was a big inspiration for this recipe.

3 cups yellow cornmeal
2¼ cups all-purpose flour
3 tablespoons low-sodium baking powder
13 beaten egg whites
6 tablespoons honey or 3 tablespoons honey and 3 tablespoons
    molasses
3 cups skim milk
Vegetable cooking spray

Preheat oven to 350 degrees. Combine the dry ingredients and mix well. Set aside. Combine the wet ingredients and mix well. Pour the wet ingredients into the dry mixture. Mix only until the dry ingredients are moistened. Do not overmix.

Spray muffin tins with vegetable cooking spray. Bake for 15 to 20 minutes. Or use a 13½ x 8¾ x 1¾-inch baking pan and bake for 25 to 30 minutes. Cut into 24 or 36 pieces.

YIELD: 24 to 36 servings

**If 24 muffins each serving contains approximately:** Calories 144, Fat .39 g, Cholesterol 0 mg, Protein 5 g, Carbohydrate 30 g, Sodium 37 mg, Calories from fat 2%

**Allowances:** 1½ starches + ⅛ protein + ⅛ dairy

**If 36 muffins each serving contains approximately:** Calories 96, Fat .26 g, Cholesterol 0 mg, Protein 3 g, Carbohydrate 20 g, Sodium 24 mg, Calories from fat 2%

**Allowances:** 1 starch + ¹⁄₁₀ protein + ¹⁄₁₂ dairy

# BASIC TOMATO SAUCE

This is a simple yet delicious tomato sauce to use with any pasta.

I carrot, diced
I onion, diced
5 garlic cloves, sliced
I tablespoon extra virgin olive oil
2 8-ounce cans tomatoes, no salt
I cup chopped basil

Sauté carrot, onion, and garlic in olive oil until soft. Crush tomatoes with hands or in food processor and add to vegetables. Simmer over low heat for 30 to 40 minutes. Add basil and serve or store.

YIELD: 8 servings (4 ounces per serving)

**Each serving contains approximately:** Calories 42, Fat calories 17, Fat 1.8 g, Saturated fat 0 g, Cholesterol 0 mg, Protein 1.8 g, Carbohydrate 6 g, Dietary fiber 1 g, Sodium 9.9 mg, Calories from fat 40%, Calories from saturated fat 0%

**Allowances:** ⅙ fat + ¾ vegetable

# CHESTNUT CORNBREAD CRANBERRY STUFFING

This stuffing is so rich, it works as a meal. It's absolutely delicious for breakfast, lunch, or dinner.

2 tablespoons extra virgin olive oil
2 green apples, peeled, cored, and chopped
I red apple, medium
I onion, chopped
¼ cup dry white wine
6 ounces dried cranberries
I teaspoon black pepper
I cup *Vegetable Stock* (p. 198) or canned chicken stock, no salt added
I pound textured vegetable protein (TVP)
I 8-ounce jar chestnuts
½ pound *Kitty's Cornbread* (p. 192), crumbled
Pinch red pepper flakes
I ounce Parmesan cheese, grated

Preheat oven to 400 degrees F.

Bring a sauté pan to medium heat with 1 tablespoon oil, then add the apples and onion and cook over a medium-low heat for 10 minutes to soften. Add the wine, cranberries, and pepper and simmer for about 5 minutes. Take off the heat and allow the mixture to cool.

Reconstitute the TVP by pouring *Vegetable Stock* over it and letting it absorb fluid for 10 minutes before draining and reserving the stock for later use.

In a large sauté pan over medium high heat, add 1 tablespoon olive oil and strained TVP.

In a medium bowl toss together the fruit and onion mixture, the strained TVP, the chestnuts, the cornbread, and the red pepper flakes.

Add the reserved *Vegetable Stock*, and ¾ of the Parmesan; mix together. Gently place into a lightly oiled 8½ x 8½–inch glass Pyrex baking dish and top with the remaining Parmesan. Place in middle rack and bake until top is golden brown, 45 minutes to 1 hour.

YIELD: 12 servings

**Each serving contains approximately:** Calories 288, Fat calories 28, Fat 3 g, Saturated Fat 0.5 g, Cholesterol 7 mg, Protein 24 g, Carbohydrates 41 g, Dietary Fiber 9 g, Sodium 129 mg, Calories from fat 10%, Calories from saturated fat 2%

**Allowances:** ½ fat + 1 starch + 3⅝ proteins + ½ fruit

# KITTY'S LOWEST SODIUM SOY SAUCE SUBSTITUTE AND DIP

This sauce can be used wherever you normally use soy sauce—but with much less sodium. Check out the *Sprout-Packed Spring Rolls* (page 205) with this soy sauce dip!

1 cube vegetable bouillon (Rapunzel's Vegan Vegetable Bouillon has
    130 mg sodium)
1 tablespoon dark or blackstrap molasses
⅛ teaspoon freshly ground black pepper
4 tablespoons apple cider vinegar
1 teaspoon toasted sesame oil
2 tablespoons garlic, minced
2 tablespoons sesame seeds, toasted
Red pepper flakes, if desired
1½ tablespoons cornstarch
3 tablespoons cilantro, freshly chopped

Bring 1½ cups of water to a boil and add all of the remaining ingredients except the cornstarch and cilantro. Dissolve the cornstarch in a few tablespoons of cold water before adding to the mixture. Simmer for a minute or two, until slightly thickened. Add cilantro just before serving.

YIELD: Makes approximately 2 cups, 32 servings (1 tablespoon per serving)

**Each serving contains approximately:** Calories 13, Fat calories 5.4, Fat 0.6 g, Saturated fat 0 g, Cholesterol 0 mg, Protein 0.2 g, Carbohydrate 1 g, Dietary fiber 0 g, Sodium 9 mg, Calories from fat 42%, Calories from saturated fat 0%

# BALSAMIC DRESSING

Nothing makes a salad more interesting than the pungent flavors of balsamic dressing.

2½ cups balsamic vinegar
1 teaspoon olive oil
6 ounces orange juice
1 tablespoon garlic, chopped
1 tablespoon basil

Place all ingredients in a blender with ½ cup water and puree about 20 seconds.

YIELD: Makes 3½ cups, 30 servings (2 tablespoons per serving)

**Each serving contains approximately:** Calories 18, Fat calories 2, Fat 0.2 g, Saturated fat 0 g, Cholesterol 0 mg, Protein 0 g, Carbohydrate 4 g, Dietary fiber 0 g, Sodium 5 mg, Calories from fat 11%, Calories from saturated fat 0%

# FISH SAUCE (WITH PASTA)

This fish sauce adds great flavor to basic starches such as polenta and pasta (recipe below), and works with egg dishes too. Try it in a frittata. For a pasta dish with great fish flavor and protein, this recipe is quick and easy.

1 tablespoon extra virgin olive oil
4 garlic cloves, sliced
3 tablespoons Italian parsley, chopped
20 sage leaves, freshly chopped
1 pound mixed fresh fish, such as orange roughy, sea bass, tuna, and halibut, finely diced (about the size of a large pea)
2 ounces brandy (100 proof)
28 ounces canned tomatoes, no salt added
2 tablespoons evaporated skim milk
Freshly ground black pepper, to taste
1 pound penne pasta (or any type you like)

Heat water for pasta in large pot.

Heat oil in a large skillet over medium heat. Add the garlic, parsley, and sage, and cook for 1 minute. Add the fish, cook less than 1 minute. Add the brandy and cook until it is almost reduced. Stir tomatoes through a food mill or chop as small as desired. Stir in the tomatoes and evaporated skim milk and season. Cook for 5 minutes.

Meanwhile, cook the pasta as directed, drain, and add the sauce.

YIELD: 8 servings

**Each serving contains approximately:** Calories 335, Fat calories 41, Fat 4.5 g, Saturated fat 1 g, Cholesterol 22 g, Protein 21 g, Carbohydrates 48 g, Dietary fiber 3 g, Sodium 72 mg, Omega-3 fatty acids 0.5 g, Calories from fat 12%, Calories from saturated fat 3%

**Allowances:** ⅜ fat + 1½ proteins + 2¾ starches + 1 vegetable

# VEGETABLE STOCK

A good vegetable stock can be used for many dishes, including soups, vegetable purees, and flavorful extra fluid for any sauté.

10–20 cups vegetable scraps saved in a plastic bag in the freezer; a
    good blend would include: skins, peelings, and/or ends from
    potatoes, onions, carrots, celery, tomatoes, and garlic
Stems from asparagus, greens, lettuce, mushrooms, parsley, etc.
Bay leaf, freshly ground black pepper, or fresh herbs, as desired
Water to cover

If you have not been saving vegetable scraps, add 2 gallons of water to:

4 large unpeeled potatoes, quartered
4 large carrots, peeled and thickly sliced
2 celery stalks, chopped
2 large onions, peeled, quartered, and sliced
1½ cups fresh corn kernels (3 ears)
1 pound mushroom stems, trimmed
1 apple, seeded and quartered
1 pear, seeded and quartered
5 heads of garlic, cut in half horizontally
6 bay leaves
25 peppercorns
1 teaspoon each chopped fresh basil, thyme, tarragon, oregano,
    parsley, and chives

Place all ingredients in a large pot and simmer for 1 to 2 hours. Pour through a colander or sieve and discard vegetable solids. The stock can be frozen in quart containers for future use as soup stock or frozen in ice cube trays for smaller needs such as stir-frying (use 1 or 2 cubes instead of oil).

The nutritional analysis is negligible for calories and fat. Sodium could be excessive if many high-sodium vegetables such as green leafy vegetables and tomatoes are used.

# RACHELLE'S MINUTE DIP

Enjoy this with raw vegetables as a dip or a topping. The roasted salsa makes this fiery and delicious, and the beans pack a soluble fiber punch.

2 teaspoons canola oil
1 onion, medium, chopped
1 15-ounce can black beans (Eden Foods)*
1 15-ounce can kidney beans (Eden Foods)*
1 cup rice, cooked
½ cup roasted salsa

* An entire can of these beans has 21 g of fiber.

Add oil to a heated Dutch oven or large skillet. Sauté onions for a few minutes over medium heat. Add all the remaining ingredients and bring to a gentle simmer. Cook for a few minutes to allow the flavors to mingle. Transfer to a food processor and blend to desired consistency. Add water if necessary to thin. Reseason to suit your taste. Enjoy!

YIELD: 12 servings (½ cup per serving)

**Each serving contains approximately:** Calories 89, Fat calories 7, Fat 0.8 g, Saturated fat 0 g, Cholesterol 0 mg, Protein 5 g, Carbohydrate 16 g, Dietary fiber 6 g, Sodium 32 mg, Calories from fat 8%, Calories from saturated fat 0%

**Allowances:** ⅛ fat + 1 starch + ¼ vegetable

# RACHELLE'S GODDESS DRESSING FOR NATALIE

This salad dressing is a winner!

½ cup vanilla soy milk, silk
⅓ cup cottage cheese, low-fat
¼ cup buttermilk, low-fat
⅖ block lite silken tofu (Nasoya brand)
⅓ cup cucumber, long, cut into large pieces
⅓ cup zucchini, cut into large pieces
1 scallion (green onion)
½ shallot, peeled and cut into thin slices
1 teaspoon dill, dried
2–3 dashes white pepper
¼ teaspoons tarragon, dried
Ground black pepper, to taste
¼ teaspoon garlic powder

Place all the ingredients into a food processor or blender and mix until nice and smooth. Reseason to taste.

YIELD: Makes 3 cups, 12 servings (¼ cup per serving)

**Each serving contains approximately:** Calories 21, Fat calories 4.5, Fat 0.5 g, Saturated fat 0 g, Cholesterol 1 mg, Protein 2 g, Carbohydrate 3 g, Dietary fiber 0 g, Sodium 49 mg, Calories from fat 21%, Calories from saturated fat 0%

**Allowances:** ½₀ dairy + ¼ protein + ⅛ vegetable

# GINGER CARROT DRESSING

Our much-appreciated intern, Kym Stork, paired with her dear friend Kerry Macaulay to adapt this recipe from their favorite sushi restaurant—Hello Sushi—in Saginaw, Michigan.

2 cups carrots, cooked

1 cup shallots, chopped

2 ounces gingerroot, sliced

¾ cup canola oil

½ cup Nakano Natural Rice Vinegar

½ cup Kitty's Lowest Sodium Soy Sauce Substitute

In a food processor or blender, puree the carrots, shallots, gingerroot, canola oil, and rice vinegar. Add the prepared soy sauce substitute. Blend until smooth.

Serve over any salad. Refrigerate leftovers in an air-tight container.

YIELD: 3½ cups (56 tablespoons)

**Each serving contains approximately:** Calories 33, Fat calories 28, Fat 3 g, Saturated fat 0.3 g, Cholesterol 0 mg, Protein 0.1 g, Carbohydrates 1.6 g, Dietary fiber 1.2 g, Sodium 4.8 mg, Calories from fat 82%, Calories from saturated fat 8%

**Allowances:** ½ fat + ½ vegetable

# APPETIZERS

Meant to tease the appetite, these flavorful appetizers are so delicious they can make a great meal!

## BRUSCHETTA WITH WHITE BEANS AND ANCHOVY

This bruschetta recipe is creamy and delicious. The sage gives it a special, nuanced flavor that complements the anchovy taste.

8 half-inch-thick slices of crusty Tuscan Bread (p. 191)
1 tablespoon extra virgin olive oil
1 15-ounce can cannellini beans, no salt added
2 anchovy fillets, chopped
3 garlic cloves, chopped
10 sage leaves, freshly chopped (or 1 teaspoon dried)
Freshly ground pepper to taste

Toast the bread.

Rinse the beans in a strainer under running water. Place washed beans in a dish and mash half of them with a fork.

Heat the olive oil, anchovies, garlic, and sage and cook, stirring, until the garlic begins to color, about 1 minute. Add the beans, season with pepper, and cook 3 minutes. Place over the toasted bread and serve.

YIELD: 8 servings

**Each serving contains approximately:** Calories 152, Fat calories 24, Fat 2.6 g, Saturated fat 1 g, Cholesterol 1 mg, Protein 6 g, Carbohydrate 26 g, Dietary fiber 3 g, Sodium 59 mg, Calories from fat 16%, Calories from saturated fat 6%

**Allowances:** ⅜ fat + 1½ starches + ⅛ protein

# TOMATO BASIL BRUSCHETTA

This is a classic bruschetta—simple to make and absolutely delicious.

2 red ripe tomatoes, seeded, finely chopped
4 basil leaves
2 garlic cloves, thinly sliced
2 teaspoons extra virgin olive oil
1 tablespoon balsamic vinegar
Freshly ground black pepper to taste
4 pieces Toufayan Pita Bread, no salt added (see Appendix A),
    toasted

Combine all ingredients except bread. Spoon the mixture onto the bread.

YIELD: 4 servings

**Each serving contains approximately:** Calories 69, Fat calories 23, Fat 3 g, Saturated fat 0 g, Cholesterol 0 mg, Protein 4 g, Carbohydrate 21 g, Fiber 1 g, Sodium 7 mg, Calories from fat 33%, Calories from saturated fat 0%

**Allowances:** ½ fat + ½ starch + ½ vegetable

# KALE BRUSCHETTA

This toasty treat is for those who love greens—it's loaded with both flavor and antioxidants.

4 garlic cloves, sliced
1 tablespoon extra virgin olive oil
8 cups kale, chopped and rinsed but not dried
Red pepper flakes, 1 or 2 pinches

4 slices Tuscan Bread (p. 191), or any no-salt Italian bread
¼ cup fat-free Parmesan cheese, grated

In a large pan sauté the garlic slices in olive oil over medium heat.
Add the kale and red pepper all at once and stir. Cover the pan and
allow the kale to cook until soft, about 12 minutes.

Grill or toast the bread and then rub with raw garlic. Top each
slice with a large spoonful of the kale mixture. Sprinkle Parmesan
over each portion.

YIELD: 4 servings

**Each serving contains approximately:** Calories 172, Fat calories 47, Fat 5.2 g, Saturated fat 0.8 g,
Cholesterol 0 mg, Protein 8 g, Carbohydrate 24 g, Dietary fiber 3 g, Sodium 144 mg, Calories from
fat 27%, Calories from saturated fat 4%

**Allowances:** ¾ fat + 1 starch + ¼ protein + 2 vegetables

# MACKEREL BRUSCHETTA

If you like the taste of this strong, omega-3–packed fish, you will enjoy it as a topping on bruschetta or toasted pita bread. You could also
try this using canned salmon or tuna.

I 15-ounce can cannellini beans, no salt added, rinsed and drained
2 4½-ounce cans cooked mackerel, in water, no salt added (see
    Appendix A)
I tablespoon extra virgin olive oil
4 tablespoons vinegar, your favorite
I red onion, chopped
½ teaspoon red pepper flakes
4 tablespoons basil leaves, chopped, or rosemary or parsley
4 garlic cloves, sliced
Ground pepper
8 pieces no-salt-added pita bread, toasted

Combine all ingredients except bread, seasoning with pepper to taste. Spoon some of the mixture onto the bread. Serve immediately.

YIELD: 8 servings

**Each serving contains approximately:** Calories 152, Fat calories 43, Fat 5 g, Saturated fat 2 g, Cholesterol 18 mg, Protein 14 g, Carbohydrate 27 g, Dietary fiber 3 g, Sodium 66 mg, Omega-3 fatty acids 0.4 g, Calories from fat 28%, Calories from saturated fat 10%

**Allowances:** ⅜ fat + ½ protein + 1½ starches + ⅙ vegetable

# SPROUT-PACKED SPRING ROLLS

My love for spring rolls has been inspired by my sister-in-law, Nancy, and my Korean friend Chung. Every year I visit my son's class at school to demonstrate how to make these rolls, and it always amazes me how adventurous—and healthy—kids become when empowered to create their own spring rolls.

6 scallions, roots removed, white plus 3 inches of green, finely
    chopped
9 cups baby greens, chopped
I cup cilantro, chopped
I cup fresh basil, chopped (preferably Thai or lemon basil)
2 organic carrots, coarsely shredded
8 ounces-weight firm tofu, cut into ¼-inch-wide strips
I 12-ounce package of grape tomatoes, sliced in half
4 cups sprouts (such as alfalfa, red clover, and broccoli sprouts)
24 spring roll wrappers (found in Asian food store or supermarket's
    Asian food aisle)
2 ounces dried bean thread noodles, thin, cooked (place in boiling
    water and take off the burner; strain in a few minutes when
    desired tenderness is reached), or I cup cooked brown rice

¼ cup roasted unsalted sunflower seeds
Very warm water, preferably spring or filtered

Wash and prep the first eight ingredients while "cooking" bean thread noodles or brown rice. Fill a large, wide bowl with hot water for dipping spring roll wrappers to soften to desired flexibility. A trial run or two is the best way to learn how long to dip your spring roll wrappers in the bowl of warm water to get them to soften just the right amount. You simply need to feel the texture of the wrapper softening enough to become elastic-like, yet not too much, or it will tear and not secure your wonderful filler ingredients. It is always easier to under-soak it; then if it needs a little more softening, you can simply add a little hot water on top of the wrapper (on a cutting board) and gently rub it until desired consistency is reached. Spring roll wrappers can be rolled tighter if they are placed on a wet kitchen towel placed on a cutting board.

Obviously, the potential for filler ingredients is limited only by your imagination! We prefer the many dark orange, red, and green vegetables and sprouts listed above because they are loaded with vitamins A, C, folic acid, potassium, and enzymes . . . which inspire health and prevent disease. Tofu is high in protein and often contains calcium; look at the ingredients list and buy the kind that contains calcium chloride (nigari) as the natural coagulant.

The spring rolls are great dipped in a low-sodium soy/toasted sesame seed oil/garlic/ginger sauce, a peanut sauce, a sweet and sour sauce (a sweet ginger chili sold at ricedietstore.com), or lemon tahini dressing.

YIELD: 24 servings (one spring roll per serving; 2 to 3 rolls make a nice entrée)

**Each serving contains approximately:** Calories 104, Fat calories 15, Fat 1.7 g, Saturated fat 0 g, Cholesterol 0 mg, Protein 5 g, Carbohydrate 20 g, Dietary fiber 2 g, Sodium 138 mg, Calories from fat 14%, Calories from saturated fat 0%

**Allowances:** ⅙ fat + ¾ starch + ⅒ protein + 1 vegetable

# SALADS AND SIDES

Many of these dishes can function as vegetable sides or salads, as well as light meals.

## PEPERONATA

A great side vegetable or a topping for bread or toast (bruschetta).

5 bell peppers (large red or yellow), seeded and sliced
1 onion, sliced
1 tablespoon extra virgin olive oil
2 tomatoes, diced
Black pepper to taste
¼ cup red wine vinegar

Sauté peppers and onion in olive oil over medium heat until soft. Add the tomatoes, season with black pepper, and cook 5 minutes. Add the vinegar, and cook and stir until the vinegar is reduced. Season with pepper.

YIELD: 6 servings

**Each serving contains approximately:** Calories 78, Fat calories 26, Fat 3 g, Saturated fat 0 g, Protein 2 g, Carbohydrate 13 g, Dietary fiber 4 g, Cholesterol 0 mg, Sodium 10 mg, Calories from fat 33%, Calories from saturated fat 0%

**Allowances:** ½ fat + 1⅗ vegetables

# ASPARAGUS-SPINACH SALAD

A salad loaded with antioxidants and delicious to boot!

20 asparagus spears, boiled and cooled, then cut into 2-inch pieces
¼ cup red onion, cubed
¼ cup tomatoes, cubed
¼ cup cucumber, cubed
¼ cup white vinegar
I teaspoon garlic, minced
I teaspoon fresh basil
I teaspoon extra virgin olive oil
I teaspoon oregano
½ teaspoon black pepper
4 cups spinach, chopped

Combine ingredients (except for spinach) in a bowl and refrigerate at least 45 minutes. Just before serving, plate spinach and top with chilled mixture.

YIELD: Makes 2 cups, 4 servings (½ cup per serving)

**Each serving contains approximately:** Calories 52, Fat calories 18, Fat 2 g, Saturated fat 0 g, Cholesterol 0 mg, Protein 3 g, Carbohydrate 8 g, Dietary fiber 3 g, Sodium 34 mg, Calories from fat 34%, Calories from saturated fat 0%

**Allowances:** ¼ fat + 1⅗ vegetables

# BABY GREENS WITH ROASTED BELL PEPPERS

A Rice House favorite as a salad or a vegetable side. If you add beans, then this becomes a meal unto itself.

½ cup red bell pepper, sliced
½ cup green bell pepper, sliced
½ cup yellow pepper, sliced
½ cup yellow onion, sliced
I teaspoon extra virgin olive oil
I tablespoon garlic, minced
I teaspoon black pepper
I teaspoon oregano
¼ cup balsamic vinegar
8 cups mixed greens

Preheat oven to 350 degrees F. Lightly toss peppers, onions, olive oil, garlic, and spices, then spread into a 2-inch-deep baking pan. Cover and bake for 20 minutes. Pour mixture into a bowl, add vinegar, and toss. Refrigerate at least 45 minutes to allow flavors to combine. Just before serving, plate mixed greens and top with pepper mixture.

YIELD: 6 servings

**Each serving contains approximately:** Calories 36, Fat calories 9, Fat 1 g, Saturated fat 0 g, Cholesterol 0 mg, Protein 1 g, Carbohydrate 7 g, Dietary fiber 1 g, Sodium 4 mg, Calories from fat 25%, Calories from saturated fat 0 %

**Allowances:** ⅙ fat + 1⅙ vegetables

# CHESS'S ROASTED ARTICHOKE SALAD

Chess, at age eight, discovered this crunchy, tasty salad all on his own, and now it's a Rosati favorite. He said it best: "I think this is the best salad I have ever eaten!" It is obviously quick and easy, too, if you have roasted artichokes and peppers already on hand.

4 medium roasted artichokes, quartered (*Roasted Artichokes alla Rosati,* p. 243)
Juice of 4 lemons
1 tablespoon extra virgin olive oil
¼ cup crumbled goat or sheep cheese (heart patients could omit)
1 cup celery, diced
¾ red onion, thinly sliced
2 roasted peppers, sliced or chopped
1 head endive, sliced
½ cup radicchio, julienned
1 tomato, chopped
1 carrot, shredded
¼ cup Italian parsley or cilantro, freshly chopped

Combine all the ingredients and serve, or better yet, marinate a few hours before serving.

I have a lot of favorite meals, but a few of them have these ingredients as key ones. A big, varied salad with Tuscan Bread (page 191) toasted and topped with roasted peppers and/or artichokes is among them!

YIELD: 4 servings

**Each serving contains approximately:**

*With cheese:* Calories 185, Fat calories 49, Fat 5.4 g, Saturated Fat 1.4g, Cholesterol 2 mg, Protein 8 g, Carbohydrate 33 g, Dietary fiber 13 g, Sodium 216 mg, Calories from fat 26%, Calories from saturated fat 7%

*Without cheese:* Calories 172, Fat calories 40, Fat 4.4 g, Saturated Fat 0.7 g, Cholesterol 0 mg, Protein 7.5 g, Carbohydrate 32 g, Dietary fiber 13 g, Sodium 192 mg, Calories from fat 23%, Calories from saturated fat 4%

**Allowances:** 1 fat + 5½ vegetables + ⅒ protein

# BARBARA CHAIKEN'S FAVORITE SALAD

Here is Barbara's absolute favorite recipe for salad. Every ingredient is optional, but I use all of them. The amount of each ingredient depends on the size of the salad. She makes a huge amount and portions out what she wants at each meal. If you don't put the dressing on, it lasts for 4 days.

15 ounces chicken, cooked, without skin or bones
2 cups romaine
1 cup carrots
1 cup celery
1 cup bell pepper, green, red, yellow, or orange
1 cup red cabbage
1 cup jicama
1 cup cucumber
1 cup green onion
1 ounce black walnuts

Chop by hand or in a food processor into bite-size pieces and place all ingredients in a large bowl.

DRESSING

1 cup balsamic vinegar
2 tablespoons Dijon mustard
4 garlic cloves
1 tomato
1 large egg white, microwaved (with a cover)

Blend all ingredients in a blender. Use on salad before eating.

VARIATION: In addition, you may want to add a pinch each of basil, oregano, rosemary, and/or parsley to give the dressing a special zing.

NOTE: A little of the dressing goes a long way. If too strong, add a little water.

YIELD: 5 servings

**Each serving contains approximately:** Calories 277, Fat calories 72, Fat 8 g, Saturated fat 1.4 g, Cholesterol 72 g, Protein 31 g, Carbohydrates 21 g, Dietary fiber 5 g, Sodium 285 mg, Calories from fat 26%, Calories from saturated fat 5%

**Allowances:** ¾ fat + 3 protein + 3 vegetables

# GRILLED SHRIMP AND CANNELLINI BEANS

This dish is a delicious way to enjoy shrimp and beans—both flavorful and nutritious.

1 8-ounce can cannellini beans, no salt added
½ onion, sliced thinly
12 medium shrimp, peeled and deveined
2 tablespoons extra virgin olive oil, plus more for brushing on
    shrimp
½ cup bread crumbs (Jaclyn's Whole Wheat Bread Crumbs are
    organic and low-sodium)
3 tablespoons Italian parsley, chopped
1 red bell pepper roasted and peeled as described in
    *Roasted Peppers*, page 239, sliced
2 tablespoons Dijon mustard, no salt added
5 tablespoons red wine vinegar
Ground black pepper, to taste

Rinse cannellini beans. Soak onion in cold water while preparing rest of salad. This step greatly reduces the harsh bite of onions.

Skewer shrimp and brush them with olive oil, and sprinkle with bread crumbs that have been mixed with 1 tablespoon of parsley. Place skewers on a hot grill and cook 2 to 3 minutes on each side. Remove shrimp from skewers and place in a bowl large enough to accommodate all ingredients.

Add drained onion slices, cannellini beans, roasted red pepper slices, and 2 tablespoons of chopped parsley and mix. Add no-salt Dijon mustard, red wine vinegar, extra virgin olive oil, and black pepper, and mix well. Enjoy.

YIELD: 4 servings

**Each serving contains approximately:** Calories 156, Fat calories 72, Omega-3 .5 g, Fat 8 g, Saturated fat 1 g, Cholesterol 32 mg, Protein 7 g, Carbohydrate 14 g, Dietary fiber 3 g, Sodium 92 mg, Calories from fat 46%, Calories from saturated fat 6%

**Allowances:** 1½ fats + ½ protein + ⅔ starch + ½ vegetable

# ITALIAN POTATO SALAD

This is a fabulous potato salad, without the mayonnaise.

4 cups potatoes, boiled and cubed
1 cup red onion, diced
¼ cup white vinegar
1 tablespoon garlic, minced
1 teaspoon extra virgin olive oil
1 pinch fresh basil
1 pinch oregano
1 pinch black pepper
1 tablespoon parsley, freshly chopped

Combine ¼ cup water and all ingredients except parsley, and refrigerate for at least 1 hour. Sprinkle with parsley and serve.

YIELD: 6 servings (½ cup per serving)

**Each serving contains approximately:** Calories 144, Fat calories 9, Fat 1 g, Saturated fat 0 g, Cholesterol 0 mg, Protein 3 g, Carbohydrate 32 g, Dietary fiber 3 g, Sodium 16 mg, Calories from fat 6%, Calories from saturated fat 0%

**Allowances:** ⅙ fat + 1⅔ starches + ⅙ vegetable

# ORIENTAL SALAD

This Rice House favorite is best served with rice, either basmati or jasmine, in keeping with the dish's Asian roots.

½ cup bean sprouts
8 grape tomatoes, halved
½ cup broccoli, blanched and diced
½ cup carrots, diced
½ cup cauliflower, blanched and diced
½ cup rice wine vinegar
¼ cup onion, diced
¼ cup lemon juice
I teaspoon garlic, minced
I pinch wasabi powder
I pinch ginger
I pinch black pepper

Wash bean sprouts and grape tomatoes well and pat dry. Mix all other ingredients (except sprouts and tomatoes) with ½ cup of water and chill for 1 hour. Place sprouts in a circle on the plate and fill the center with the refrigerated mixture. Top with grape tomatoes.

YIELD: 2 servings (1¼ cup per serving)

**Each serving contains approximately:** Calories 80, Fat calories 7.2, Fat 0.8 g, Saturated fat 0.1 g, Cholesterol 0 mg, Protein 4 g, Carbohydrate 18 g, Dietary fiber 5 g, Sodium 42 mg, Calories from fat 9%, Calories from saturated fat 1%

**Allowances:** 3 vegetables

# ITALIAN BREAD SALAD

This recipe is perfect as a starter or a summer lunch. You will be surprised how delicious this recipe is given its simplicity.

8 ounces Tuscan Bread (p. 191)
3 tomatoes, diced
1 red onion, diced
15 basil leaves, shredded
9 pitted black olives
3 tablespoons red wine vinegar
4 garlic cloves, quartered
2 tablespoons extra virgin olive oil
Freshly ground pepper, to taste
1 7-ounce can tuna, water-packed, low-sodium, drained

Break the bread into pieces and soak briefly in cold water. Squeeze the bread dry. Add the tomatoes, onion, basil, and olives.

Combine the vinegar, garlic, and olive oil and mix well. Add the dressing and several grinds of pepper to the salad with the tuna and mix gently.

YIELD: 6 servings

**Each serving contains approximately:** Calories 212, Fat calories 64, Fat 7 g, Saturated fat 1 g, Cholesterol 10 mg, Protein 13 g, Carbohydrate 24 g, Dietary fiber 2 g, Sodium 165 mg, Calories from fat 30%, Calories from saturated fat 4%

**Allowances:** 1 fat + 1 protein + 1¼ starches + ½ vegetable

# SPINACH AND MANDARIN ORANGE SALAD

This salad reminds us of summer: it's refreshing yet surprisingly substantial.

6 cups spinach, chopped
1¼ cups mandarin oranges, canned and drained
¼ cup Balsamic Dressing (page 196)
1 pinch black pepper

Plate spinach and sprinkle with oranges. Drizzle with Balsamic Dressing and serve.

YIELD: 4 servings

**Each serving contains approximately:** Calories 48, Fat calories 3, Fat 0.3 g, Saturated fat 0 g, Cholesterol 0 mg, Protein 2 g, Carbohydrate 11 g, Dietary fiber 2 g, Sodium 42 mg, Calories from fat 6%, Calories from saturated fat 0%

**Allowances:** ½ vegetable + ⅜ fruit

# TACO SALAD

Ricers love to mix the Southwestern Corn recipe (page 241) with their Taco Salad for a wonderful lunch or light dinner.

8 corn tortillas, no salt
4 cups lettuce, shredded
1½ cups tomato, diced
½ cup yellow onion, diced
¼ cup red wine vinegar
1½ tablespoons fresh cilantro, diced
1 tablespoon garlic, minced

1 tablespoon lemon juice
1 teaspoon black pepper

Preheat oven to 350 degrees F. Cut tortillas in quarters and bake 5 to 7 minutes or until crispy. Set aside with lettuce. Mix remaining ingredients in a bowl and refrigerate for at least 45 minutes. Plate lettuce and top with tomato salsa mixture, then edge plate with chips.

YIELD: 5 servings (½ cup per serving)

**Each serving contains approximately:** Calories 130, Fat calories 9, Fat 1 g, Saturated fat 0 g, Cholesterol 0 mg, Protein 4 g, Carbohydrate 29 g, Dietary fiber 4 g, Sodium 27 mg, Calories from fat 7%, Calories from saturated fat 0%

**Allowances:** 1 starch + 2 vegetables

# RACHELLE'S BARLEY AND LENTIL SALAD

This salad has great texture—both tender and chewy—and will surprise you with its flavorfulness. It is a great low-fat recipe with lots of protein and fiber. Use a ½-cup portion as a side salad or have a 1-cup portion if you eat this as the main course.

1 cup black barley, uncooked
1 cup green lentils, uncooked
5 garlic cloves, minced
1 cup red onion, chopped
1 cup celery, minced
¾ cup Italian parsley, minced
1 tablespoon olive oil
1 tablespoon sesame oil
⅓ cup lemon juice, freshly squeezed
1 tablespoon Dijon mustard

Bring the barley and 2½ cups of water to a boil in a saucepan. Reduce the heat and simmer, partially covered, until the water is absorbed and the barley is tender, approximately 45 minutes.

Bring the lentils and 2 cups of water to a boil in a saucepan. Reduce the heat and simmer, partially covered, until the water is absorbed and the lentils are tender, approximately 20 to 30 minutes.

Transfer the barley and lentils to a medium-size bowl, and stir in the garlic. When the barley and lentils have cooled, stir in the onion, celery, and parsley. It's fine to cook the barley and the lentils the night before and just take them out of the refrigerator the following day to continue the recipe. (Try adding cayenne pepper, black pepper, and a little cumin to the serving—this tastes much better the next day.)

Whisk together the olive oil, sesame oil, lemon juice, and mustard. Stir the dressing into the salad and serve at room temperature.

YIELD: 9 servings

**Each serving contains approximately:** Calories 197, Fat calories 36, Fat 4 g, Saturated fat 0.5 g, Cholesterol 0 mg, Protein 10 g, Carbohydrate 28 g, Dietary fiber 11 g, Sodium 22 mg, Calories from fat 18%, Calories from saturated fat 2%

**Allowances:** ⅔ fat + 1⅓ starches + ⅔ vegetable

# RACHELLE'S BLACK BEAN AND CORN SALAD

This is a refreshing and flavorful salad that's full of color. It tastes best chilled and keeps well in the fridge. It makes a great side dish or main course. Adjust the serving size to suit your meal needs.

¼ cup balsamic vinegar
¼ cup cider vinegar
1 tablespoon brown sugar

½ teaspoon lime juice, freshly squeezed

½ teaspoon cumin, ground

1 garlic clove, minced

1 cup corn, fresh or frozen

1 red bell pepper, medium, chopped

1 red onion, chopped

⅓ cup fresh cilantro, minced

1 15-ounce can black beans, no salt added, rinsed and drained

Mix the first six ingredients together in a saucepan. Bring to a boil and stir, then simmer for 1 to 2 minutes more to ensure sugar has dissolved. Remove from heat. Mix the remaining ingredients. Add the contents of the saucepan to the corn mixture and mix well. Cover and chill. Serve cold.

YIELD: 4 servings (1 cup per serving)

**Each serving contains approximately:** Calories 182, Fat calories 3.6, Fat 0.4 g, Saturated fat 0 g, Cholesterol 0 mg, Protein 8 g, Carbohydrate 36 g, Dietary fiber 9 g, Sodium 16 mg, Calories from fat 2%, Calories from saturated fat 0%

**Allowances:** 1⅛ starches + 1 vegetable

# RACHELLE'S FENNEL, QUINOA, ORANGE, WALNUT, AND BASIL SALAD

This recipe is adapted from Chef Andree Robert, Executive Chef, Maison Robert (Boston), and appeared in "There Is No Place Like Maison," *Cooking Light*, May 1997. "In this dish, the fresh orange and fennel marry really well with the flavor of the nutty quinoa, making for an interesting main-dish salad with many rich textures," Andree says.

3 cups quinoa, cooked
1 cup fennel bulb, chopped
3 tablespoons shallots, minced
1 teaspoon lemon rind, grated
1 teaspoon orange rind, grated
⅔ cup fresh orange juice
2 tablespoons fresh lemon juice
¼ cup fresh basil, chopped
2 teaspoons sesame oil
⅛ teaspoon pepper
2 cups orange sections
¼ cup toasted walnuts, chopped

Combine quinoa, fennel, and shallots in a large bowl; set aside. Combine lemon rind, orange rind, juices, basil, sesame oil, and pepper in a small bowl; stir well. Pour over quinoa mixture; toss well. Spoon 1 cup of salad onto each of four plates. Arrange ½ cup orange sections around each salad; sprinkle each salad with 1 tablespoon walnuts.

YIELD: 4 servings (1 cup per serving)

**Each serving contains approximately:** Calories 381, Fat calories 96, Fat 10.7 g, Saturated fat 1 g, Cholesterol 0 mg, Protein 11 g, Carbohydrate 68 g, Dietary fiber 8 g, Sodium 26 mg, Calories from fat 25%, Calories from saturated fat 2%

**Allowances:** 1½ fat + 2½ starches + ⅜ vegetable + 1⅜ fruits

# RACHELLE'S LENTIL QUINOA SALAD

Lentils are a wonderful food, naturally low in sodium, high in fiber, and high in protein. Quinoa is a grain from South America that is very versatile and a nutritional powerhouse in its own right. Together, they make a smashing duo, drenched in this sultry lime-curry vinaigrette. Because beans/grains are nutritionally dense, they also come with calories—use this dish as a modest-size main course or serve half the amount for a side dish.

1 cup lentils, uncooked
½ cup quinoa, uncooked
⅓ cup scallions, chopped

LIME-CURRY VINAIGRETTE

⅛ cup canola oil
6 tablespoons lime juice, freshly squeezed
2 tablespoons curry powder
2 tablespoons ginger, freshly grated
1 teaspoon ground coriander

Cook the lentils until tender, about 20 minutes. Drain and allow to cool. Cook the quinoa per instructions until translucent and tender. Allow to cool; there should not be any water remaining in the pot. Chop scallions; use more if you like. Place all the ingredients for the vinaigrette in a separate bowl and stir thoroughly. Adjust spices to suit your taste. Mix the lentils, quinoa, and scallions together in a large serving bowl and fold in the vinaigrette.

YIELD: 5 servings (1 cup per serving)

**Each serving contains approximately:** Calories 261, Fat calories 63, Fat 7 g, Saturated fat 0.5 g, Cholesterol 0 mg, Protein 13 g, Carbohydrate 38 g, Dietary fiber 6 g, Sodium 9 mg, Calories from fat 24%, Calories from saturated fat 2%

**Allowances:** 1½ fats + 2½ starches

# RACHELLE'S ASIAN SALAD

This is a refreshing way to use tofu for a main course at lunch. Tofu is made from soybeans and is a wonderful source of protein and calcium.

1 tablespoon sesame oil
1 teaspoon ginger juice
2 teaspoons low-sodium Worcestershire sauce
1 teaspoon maple syrup
1 tablespoon toasted sesame seeds
2 tablespoons orange juice
3/5 block tofu, firm style
Cooking oil spray
1 cup shiitake mushrooms, sliced
3 cups iceberg lettuce, thinly sliced
3 large scallions, thinly sliced
2/3 cup mandarin orange slices

Mix the sesame oil, ginger juice, Worcestershire sauce, maple syrup, sesame seeds, and orange juice in a large measuring cup.

Cut off 3/5 of the tofu block and return the unused portion to the refrigerator for another meal. Gently cut the tofu into small cubes. Add the tofu to the marinade and cover. Marinate overnight in the refrigerator, tossing the tofu gently whenever you think about it.

Coat a nonstick frying pan lightly with cooking oil spray. Fry tofu cubes until nice and crispy on the outside. Save the marinade. Set aside cooked tofu on a plate. Add mushrooms to the pan and sauté for a few minutes, then remove from heat.

Serve each person ½ of the tofu and the mushrooms atop a bed of lettuce. Drizzle remaining marinade equally over each portion. Scatter ½ of the scallions over each serving as a garnish. Complete the plate with the mandarin orange slices.

YIELD: 2 servings

**Each serving contains approximately:** Calories 374, Fat calories 144, Fat 16 g, Saturated fat 2.5 g, Cholesterol 0 mg, Protein 17 g, Carbohydrate 22 g, Dietary fiber 6 g, Sodium 53 mg, Calories from fat 39%, Calories from saturated fat 6%

**Allowances:** 2 fats + 1⅔ proteins + 2⅓ vegetables + 1 fruit

# QUINOA VEGGIE SALAD

Quinoa is both tasty and nutritious and makes this salad a protein-packed winner. Try it with a cold bean salad or a dip, or served on a bed of lettuce as a light lunch or dinner.

1½ cups quinoa
½ cup dried cherries or raisins
4 tablespoons lime or lemon juice, freshly squeezed
1 tablespoon orange juice
1 cup orange bell pepper, chopped
1 cup yellow bell pepper, chopped
½ cup scallions, chopped
½ cup cilantro or Italian parsley, freshly chopped
1 tomato, diced
Freshly ground black pepper or gourmet blend of red, green,
    and black peppercorns, to taste

Rinse quinoa with hot water until water runs clear. Bring 3½ cups of water to a boil. Pour ½ cup boiling water over cherries or raisins and set aside for 15 minutes. Add rinsed quinoa to remaining boiling water and simmer, covered, for 15 minutes, then remove from heat and let sit for 5 minutes. Fluff up with a fork, then stir in the cherries and other ingredients.

YIELD: 15 servings

**Each serving contains approximately:** Calories 91, Fat calories 9, Fat 1 g, Saturated fat 0 g, Cholesterol 0 mg, Protein 3 g, Carbohydrate 20 g, Dietary fiber 2 g, Sodium 7 mg, Calories from fat 10%, Calories from saturated fat 0%

**Allowances:** ⅔ starch + ⅓ vegetable + ⅓ fruit

# SHIITAKE SLAW

Coleslaw with a twist!

1 teaspoon extra virgin olive oil
1 tablespoon garlic, minced
1¼ cups shiitake mushrooms, stems removed and julienned
1 teaspoon dry mustard
1 teaspoon dill
3 cups red cabbage, julienned
¼ cup red onion, diced
¼ cup white wine vinegar
1 teaspoon black pepper

In a small pot, sauté garlic and mushrooms in olive oil over low-medium heat until lightly browned. Add ¼ cup water, mustard, and dill, and sauté 2 to 3 minutes. Cover and remove from heat. Combine cabbage, onion, and vinegar in a mixing bowl. Stir in mushroom sauté and black pepper. Refrigerate at least 1 hour before serving.

YIELD: 3 servings (1 cup per serving)

**Each serving contains approximately:** Calories 97, Fat calories 18, Fat 2 g, Saturated fat 0 g, Cholesterol 0 mg, Protein 3 g, Carbohydrate 19 g, Dietary fiber 3 g, Sodium 12 mg, Calories from fat 19%, Calories from saturated fat 0%

**Allowances:** ⅓ fat + 3¼ vegetables

# SUSAN LEVY'S WILD RICE SALAD

In addition to managing the Rice Diet Store, Susan leads yoga, coteaches olive oil and vinegar tastings, and rivals cooking school with dishes like this!

½ cup wild rice

½ pound asparagus, roasted

2 teaspoons olive oil

1 red pepper, roasted

4 halves sun-dried tomatoes

2 tablespoons pine nuts

1½ teaspoons red wine vinegar

½ teaspoon Dijon mustard, no salt added

2 teaspoons fresh basil, chopped

Black pepper, to taste

Simmer rice in 1½ cups of water for 25 to 50 minutes. I'd suggest 40 minutes. Preheat oven to 400 degrees F.

Cut asparagus into 1-inch lengths, toss with ½ teaspoon olive oil, and roast for 5 to 7 minutes. Cut pepper into four segments and roast for 30 minutes. Peel the pepper when cool and cut into bite-size pieces.

Reconstitute tomatoes in hot water and chop. Toast pine nuts until lightly browned. Drain rice and mix with vegetables and nuts.

Mix vinegar with mustard and chopped basil. Whisk 1½ teaspoons oil into vinegar. Add black pepper to taste.

Toss salad and chill for a few hours to cool ingredients and let flavors meld.

YIELD: 2 servings

**Each serving contains approximately:** Calories 293, Fat calories 90, Fat 11 g, Saturated fat 1 g, Cholesterol 0 mg, Protein 10 g, Carbohydrate 41 g, Dietary fiber 7 g, Sodium 54 mg, Calories from fat 31%, Calories from saturated fat 3%

**Allowances:** 2 fats + 1⅞ starches + 2 vegetables

# BAKED EGGPLANT SLICES

Eggplant is a vegetable that can stand alone as a meal or serve as a great side. This dish will give any lasagne a run for its money!

3 whole bell peppers, chopped
1 cup yellow onion, chopped
1 tablespoon garlic cloves, chopped
½ cup grits, uncooked
2 teaspoons extra virgin olive oil
1½ large eggplants, peeled and cut into 2-inch strips

Preheat oven to 450 degrees F. Clean, seed, and chop peppers. Chop onions and garlic as well. Puree these ingredients in a blender, adding a little water if necessary. Cook grits according to package directions. Mix with puree to create a batter and set aside. Coat a cookie sheet lightly with olive oil. Dip eggplant in batter, place on sheet, and bake for 50 minutes or until browned.

YIELD: 4 servings

**Each serving contains approximately:** Calories 180, Fat calories 27, Fat 3 g, Saturated fat 0.5 g, Cholesterol 0 mg, Protein 5 g, Carbohydrate 36 g, Dietary fiber 6 g, Sodium 14 mg, Calories from fat 15%, Calories from saturated fat 3%

**Allowances:** ½ fat + ½ starch + 4 vegetables

# BLACK BEANS AND GARLIC

Beans are both hearty and full of flavor. Mix this dish with a green salad and call it a meal.

1½ cups black beans
1 cup yellow onion, diced

1 tablespoon garlic, minced
½ teaspoon black pepper
½ teaspoon oregano
½ teaspoon basil
2 bay leaves

Soak beans for at least 4 hours, preferably rinsing a few times with fresh water. Use 3 parts water to one part beans to soak; use bottled water if tap water is hard. Soak, and later cook, in a pot at least 4 times the volume of the beans, as the beans will double in size while soaking, and the water will bubble up ⅓ higher than the beans. Strain, rinse, and cover soaked beans with 6 cups fresh water. Boil for 5 minutes, reduce heat to medium, and simmer for 45 minutes or until slightly tender. Reduce heat, add remaining ingredients, and simmer for 40 minutes to 1 hour.

YIELD: 9 servings (½ cup per serving)

**Each serving contains approximately:** Calories 117, Fat calories 5, Fat 0.5 g, Saturated fat 0 g, Cholesterol 0 mg, Protein 7 g, Carbohydrate 23 g, Dietary fiber 7 g, Sodium 3 mg, Calories from fat 4%, Calories from saturated fat 0%

**Allowances:** 1¼ starches + ⅒ vegetable

# BOK CHOY

This Asian vegetable is a head turner at the Rice House. Chef J.R. likes to serve it with potatoes. Keep the juice from the dish and use it as a topping for rice, potatoes, or pasta.

1 teaspoon extra virgin olive oil
½ cup leek, diced
3 ounces apple juice
8 cups bok choy, coarsely chopped
¼ cup tomato puree, no salt added

Heat olive oil in a large frying pan on medium heat. Then add leeks and sauté until lightly browned. Add apple juice and simmer 2 to 3 minutes. Add bok choy, cook another 3 to 5 minutes; add tomato puree and remove from heat. Stir well, cover, and let set for 3 minutes before serving.

YIELD: 7 servings (½ cup per serving)

**Each serving contains approximately:** Calories 27, Fat calories 9, Fat 1 g, Saturated fat 0 g, Cholesterol 0 mg, Protein 1 g, Carbohydrate 4 g, Dietary fiber 1 g, Sodium 54 mg, Calories from fat 33%, Calories from saturated fat 0%

**Allowances:** ½ fat + ⅖ vegetable

# BRAISED FENNEL

The subtle licorice taste of fennel is mellowed in the braising, making this savory dish a great side with pasta. You may be surprised by how delicious this is. Kitty, who previously said she did not like fennel, sure was!

6 fennel bulbs, quartered
2 tablespoons extra virgin olive oil
3 garlic cloves
3 anchovy fillets, chopped
½ teaspoon red pepper flakes

Steam fennel until tender, drain, and cut into mouth-sized pieces.

Heat the oil, the garlic, anchovies, and pepper flakes for 3 minutes. Add the fennel and continue cooking, stirring to coat the fennel until fennel is warm.

YIELD: 6 servings

**Each serving contains approximately:** Calories 122, Fat calories 49, Fat 5.4 g, Saturated fat 0.7 g, Cholesterol 1.7 mg, Protein 4 g, Carbohydrate 18 g, Dietary fiber 7 g, Sodium 195 mg, Calories from fat 39%, Calories from saturated fat 5%

**Allowances:** 1 fat + ⅙ protein + 3⅗ vegetables

# BROCCOLI RABE

Another Rice House favorite!

1 tablespoon extra virgin olive oil
1 pound broccoli rabe, broccolini, or broccoli spears, cut into pieces
5 garlic cloves, chopped
1 cup dry white wine
1 tablespoon red chili flakes
1 lemon and 1 orange, zested

Heat the olive oil and add the broccoli rabe and garlic and cook, tossing regularly, for 8 to 10 minutes, until tender. Use the wine to slow the cooking down if the garlic begins to brown. When the broccoli rabe is tender, add the chili flakes and zests.

YIELD: 4 servings

**Each serving contains approximately:** Calories 107, Fat calories 38, Fat 4 g, Saturated fat 0 g, Cholesterol 0 mg, Protein 4 g, Carbohydrate 9 g, Dietary fiber 7 g, Sodium 34 mg, Calories from fat 36%, Calories from saturated fat 8%

**Allowances:** ¾ fat + 2½ vegetables

# BRUSSELS SPROUTS, ONIONS, AND CHESTNUTS

A great dish in the fall or winter. The caramelized onions are a slice of heaven!

2½ pounds Brussels sprouts
3 red onions, medium, thinly sliced
2 tablespoons extra virgin olive oil
6 garlic cloves, sliced
10 unsalted sun-dried tomatoes, chopped
8 ounces chestnuts, roughly chopped

Clean and steam Brussels sprouts for 5 to 7 minutes. Allow to cool and cut in half.

Sauté onion slices in 1 tablespoon of extra virgin olive oil over high heat until caramelized. Add garlic and cook one minute more. Place onions in a bowl. Sauté Brussels sprout halves in 1 tablespoon of extra virgin olive oil. Cook until caramelized. Add onions, sun-dried tomatoes, and chestnuts. Combine and cook 1 to 2 minutes more.

YIELD: 7 cups, 10 servings (¾ cup per serving)

**Each serving contains approximately:** Calories 109, Fat calories 30, Fat 3.3 g, Saturated fat 0.5 g, Cholesterol 0 mg, Protein 2 g, Carbohydrate 18 g, Dietary fiber 2 g, Sodium 51 mg, Calories from fat 27%, Calories from saturated fat 4%

**Allowances:** ⅖ fat + ¾ starch + 1 vegetable

# BUTTERNUT SQUASH

This is another vegetable that is abundant in the fall and early winter. Enjoy as a side or a main course with a side salad.

1 butternut squash, medium
½ teaspoon extra virgin olive oil
1–1½ cup pineapple chunks in juice
1 teaspoon pumpkin pie spice

Preheat oven to 350 degrees F. Rinse squash, cut in half lengthwise, and scoop out seeds. Place squash cut side up in a pan lightly coated with olive oil. Place the pineapple chunks and juice in squash cavity and sprinkle with pumpkin pie spice. Flip squash over carefully so that pineapple remains in cavity. Bake squash about 30 to 50 minutes or until it's soft all the way through—you should be able to pierce squash easily with a fork.

NOTE: Serve squash skin side down. Order small squash.

YIELD: 2 servings

**Each serving contains approximately:** Calories 335, Fat calories 27, Fat 3 g, Saturated fat 0 g, Cholesterol 0 mg, Protein 6 g, Carbohydrate 84 g, Dietary fiber 19 g, Sodium 27 mg, Calories from fat 8%, Calories from saturated fat 0%

**Allowances:** ¼ fat + 3 starches + ¼ fruit

# CRAZY CAULIFLOWER WITH ROASTED GARLIC

No one at the Rice House ever forgets crazy cauliflower! The crunch, the taste, and the sense of satisfaction are superb!

3 teaspoons olive oil
24 garlic cloves, peeled and cleaned
3¾ cups cauliflower florets
½ teaspoon paprika, or to taste
½ teaspoon freshly ground black pepper, or to taste
½ teaspoon onion powder, or to taste

Preheat oven to 350 degrees F. Mix 1½ teaspoons olive oil and whole garlic cloves in a 2-inch-deep baking pan. Bake until golden brown, about 25 to 45 minutes, checking every 5 to 10 minutes and stirring well. Mix all other ingredients in a large bowl. Add this mixture to the roasted garlic and mix well. Continue baking at 350 degrees F until cauliflower is tender, about 30 to 45 minutes.

YIELD: 6 servings (½ cup per serving)

**Each serving contains approximately:** Calories 57, Fat calories 24, Fat 2.7 g, Saturated fat 0.4 g, Cholesterol 0 mg, Protein 2 g, Carbohydrate 8 g, Dietary fiber 2 g, Soluble fiber 0.7 g, Sodium 43 mg, Calories from fat 42%, Calories from saturated fat 6%

**Allowances:** ½ fat + 1⅓ vegetables

# CREAMED SPINACH

This dish simply melts in your mouth. Serve it over potatoes or pasta for a full, pleasing meal.

10 cups spinach, or about 3 cups chopped
2 cups cauliflower
2 teaspoons garlic, minced
2 teaspoons olive oil
½ cup onion, diced
2 cups zucchini, diced
1 pinch basil
1 pinch oregano
1 pinch black pepper

Chop spinach in a blender or food processor and set aside. Boil cauliflower 5 to 7 minutes or until very soft and set aside. Sauté garlic in olive oil; add onions and sauté until slightly brown. Add zucchini, herbs, and pepper, and simmer 10 minutes or until zucchini is tender. Place cauliflower and sautéed mixture in a blender or food processor and puree. In the same pan, sauté spinach 3 to 5 minutes. Add puree, mix well, and serve.

YIELD: 4½ cups, 9 servings (½ cup per serving)

**Each serving contains approximately:** Calories 28, Fat calories 9, Fat 1 g, Saturated fat 0 g, Cholesterol 0 mg, Protein 1 g, Carbohydrate 4 g, Dietary fiber 1 g, Sodium 13 mg, Calories from fat 32%, Calories from saturated fat 0%

**Allowances:** ⅕ fat + ¾ vegetable

# GARLIC RED SKIN POTATOES

The simplicity of this dish matches its deliciousness. Add a little cayenne pepper if you like some kick!

18 red potatoes, small, halved
1 tablespoon olive oil
1 tablespoon oregano
1 tablespoon parsley
1 tablespoon rosemary
1 tablespoon basil, freshly chopped
1 tablespoon black pepper
1 teaspoon garlic, minced
1 teaspoon thyme

Preheat oven to 350 degrees F. Combine ingredients in a bowl making sure to coat the potatoes with the spice mixture. Lay potatoes on a cookie sheet. Use a spatula to remove any spice mixture in the bowl. Bake for 45 minutes—or longer if you like them crunchy!

YIELD: 20 servings (½ cup per serving)

**Each serving contains approximately:** Calories 127, Fat calories 7, Fat 1 g, Saturated fat 0 g, Cholesterol 0 mg, Protein 3 g, Carbohydrate 26 g, Dietary fiber 3 g, Sodium 11 mg, Calories from fat 6%, Calories from saturated fat 0%

**Allowances:** ⅒ fat + 1½ starches

# GARLIC ROASTED VEGGIES

Pair these roasted vegetables with salad, pasta, risotto, rice, or polenta to create a tasty, satisfying meal. You can also accompany them with a fish or chicken dish. It's great to always have these around for leftovers to use with pasta or in sandwiches.

3 cups button mushrooms

1 red bell pepper, chopped

1 green bell pepper, chopped

1 yellow bell pepper, chopped

½ yellow squash, diced

½ zucchini, diced

½ carrot, diced

½ cup yellow onion, diced

2 teaspoons garlic cloves, chopped

1 teaspoon olive oil

½ teaspoon dried thyme

½ teaspoon black pepper, freshly ground

Preheat oven to 375 degrees F. Mix all ingredients in 2-inch-deep pan and bake uncovered for 10 minutes. Stir, cover, and bake 15 more minutes. Mix well and serve.

YIELD: 6 servings (½ cup per serving)

**Each serving contains approximately:** Calories 46, Fat calories 9, Fat 1 g, Saturated fat 0 g, Cholesterol 0 mg, Protein 2 g, Carbohydrate 9 g, Dietary fiber 2 g, Sodium 7 mg, Calories from fat 20%, Calories from saturated fat 0%

**Allowances:** ⅙ fat + 1¾ vegetables

# GRILLED PORTOBELLO MUSHROOMS

This meaty mushroom is succulent and just as satisfying as any steak—and so much better for you. Try it served cold over baby greens as well.

6 large portobello mushroom caps
¼ cup your favorite vinegar, red wine, champagne, or balsalmic
I tablespoon garlic, minced
I teaspoon extra virgin olive oil
½ teaspoon black pepper

Grill portobellos about 2 to 3 minutes on each side. Chop mushrooms and combine with remaining ingredients and ¼ cup water.

YIELD: 6 servings (½ cup per serving)

**Each serving contains approximately:** Calories 12, Fat calories 7, Fat 0.8 g, Saturated fat 0 g, Cholesterol 0 mg, Protein 0.4 g, Carbohydrate 2 g, Dietary fiber 0 g, Sodium 0.7 mg, Calories from fat 58%, Calories from saturated fat 0%

**Allowances:** ⅙ fat + ½ vegetable

# MARINATED VEGETABLES

Ricers love this dish as both a salad and as a vegetable side. It's packed with flavor and nutrients. These vegetables are great to keep on hand for sandwiches, bruschetta toppings, or tossed into pasta or risotto. They are almost better as leftovers.

2 Italian eggplants, cut into ½-inch slices lengthwise
2 red bell peppers, sliced
2 yellow bell peppers, sliced

¼ cup extra virgin olive oil, plus more for brushing vegetables
1½ pounds zucchini, sliced
½ pound asparagus
3 carrots, peeled and sliced
2 pounds tomatoes
3 Vidalia onions, sliced
1 pound new potatoes, quartered
½ cup white wine vinegar
8 garlic cloves, minced
2 anchovies, minced
3 tablespoons oregano, chopped
Black pepper, to taste

Brush vegetables with olive oil and grill (or broil) until tender.

Combine ¼ cup olive oil, vinegar, garlic, anchovies, oregano, and pepper, and mix well. Pour the mixture over the vegetables, cover, and marinate overnight.

YIELD: 8 servings

**Each serving contains approximately:** Calories 230, Fat calories 72, Fat 8 g, Saturated fat 1 g, Cholesterol 1 mg, Protein 7 g, Carbohydrate 36 g, Dietary fiber 10 g, Sodium 72 mg, Calories from fat 31%, Calories from saturated fat 4%

**Allowances:** 1½ fats + 1 starch + 3 vegetables

# RED BELL PEPPER WITH ORZO STUFFING

These tender bell peppers are perfectly matched with orzo to give you a wonderful side or main dish. These are also a Rice House favorite. Chef J.R.'s ("the Grinch") heart melts from all the compliments he receives on the days these are served.

¾ cup orzo, cooked and drained
1 teaspoon extra virgin olive oil
1 cup red onion, diced
1 tablespoon garlic, minced
4 red bell peppers, tops removed
8 cherry tomatoes, chopped
1½ tablespoons tomato puree, no-salt added
1 tablespoon fresh basil, diced
1 teaspoon black pepper
1 teaspoon oregano
1 teaspoon honey

Preheat oven to 350 degrees F. Cook orzo according to directions on package. Sauté onions and garlic in olive oil until lightly browned. Add remaining ingredients and up to 1½ cups water, as needed, and continue to sauté for 4 to 5 minutes. Mix cooked orzo into mixture, reduce heat to low, and continue to cook until most of the moisture is gone. After allowing mixture to cool for 5 minutes, stuff peppers and place in a 2-inch-deep baking pan. Add a little water to pan, cover, and bake for 35 to 40 minutes.

YIELD: 4 servings

**Each serving contains approximately:** Calories 128, Fat calories 18, Fat 2 g, Saturated fat 0 g, Cholesterol 0 mg, Protein 8 g, Carbohydrate 20 g, Dietary fiber 3 g, Sodium 13 mg, Calories from fat 8%, Calories from saturated fat 0%

**Allowances:** ¼ fat + 1 starch + 1½ vegetables

# ROASTED PEPPERS

These are a staple at our house—on toast or pasta or a salad, they are what we call convenience food!

8 peppers, red or yellow
1 tablespoon extra virgin olive oil
3 garlic cloves, sliced
½ teaspoon black pepper
3 tablespoons balsamic vinegar
2 tablespoons parsley or basil, chopped

Brush peppers with olive oil and place under broiler for 10 to 15 minutes, until the skin is blackened, turning occasionally. Place peppers in a zip-lock bag and allow to cool. This step inspires sweating, making them easier to peel. Peel off blackened skin, slice into strips, place in medium bowl, and toss with remaining ingredients. Let mixture marinate for at least two hours. Serve as a side dish or on bruschetta.

YIELD: 8 servings

**Each serving contains approximately:** Calories 48, Fat calories 18, Fat 2 g, Saturated fat 0 g, Cholesterol 0 mg, Protein 1 g, Carbohydrate 8 g, Dietary fiber 2 g, Sodium 4 mg, Calories from fat 38%, Calories from saturated fat 0%

**Allowances:** ⅜ fat + 1⅙ vegetables

# SESAME VEGETABLES

This Asian-inspired dish is great with a side salad or another appetizer.

1 teaspoon extra virgin olive oil
1 cup yellow onions, chopped fine
3 cups zucchini, cut into 1" strips
2 cups snow pea pods, fresh
5 ounces bamboo shoots, canned, drained
5 ounces water chestnuts, canned, drained
2 tablespoons balsamic vinegar
3 tablespoons sesame seeds

Sauté the onions in olive oil. Add the zucchini and ½ cup water, cover, and sauté 2 to 3 minutes. Add the snow peas, bamboo shoots, water chestnuts, and vinegar and sauté for 4 to 5 minutes. Stir in sesame seeds, cover, and sauté on low heat 2 to 3 minutes or until vegetables reach desired tenderness.

YIELD: 11 servings (½ cup per serving)

**Each serving contains approximately:** Calories 53, Fat calories 18, Fat 2 g, Saturated fat 0 g, Cholesterol 0 mg, Protein 2 g, Carbohydrate 8 g, Dietary fiber 28 g, Sodium 10 mg, Calories from fat 34%, Calories from saturated fat 0%

**Allowances:** 2 vegetables

# SICILIAN EGGPLANT

This eggplant dish is a marvelous side to J.R.'s meatloaf or great on its own.

8 cups eggplant, peeled and cubed
1 cup red onion, chopped

½ cup tomato puree, no salt added
¼ cup balsamic vinegar
1 tablespoon garlic, chopped
½–1 teaspoon red pepper, crushed
1 teaspoon extra virgin olive oil
1 pinch black pepper

Preheat oven to 350 degrees F. Combine ingredients with ¼ cup water in a baking dish, cover, and bake 45 minutes or until eggplant reaches desired tenderness.

YIELD: 3 cups, 6 servings (½ cup per serving)

**Each serving contains approximately:** Calories 79, Fat calories 9, Fat 1 g, Saturated fat 0 g, Cholesterol 0 mg, Protein 2 g, Carbohydrate 17 g, Dietary fiber 4 g, Sodium 15 mg, Calories from fat 11%, Calories from saturated fat 0%

**Allowances:** ⅙ fat + 2¾ vegetables

# SOUTHWESTERN CORN

Mix this spicy corn dish with either the Taco Salad (page 216) or chili for a fabulous lunch or dinner.

4½ cups corn, fresh or frozen
¼ cup red onion, diced
¼ cup red pepper, diced
¼ cup green pepper, diced
¼ cup yellow pepper, diced
1 teaspoon cilantro, freshly chopped
1 teaspoon fresh basil, chopped
1 teaspoon extra virgin olive oil
1 teaspoon paprika or pinch of cayenne pepper

Boil corn for 5 to 6 minutes and strain. Add remaining ingredients and mix well.

Yield: 8 servings (½ cup per serving)

**Each serving contains approximately:** Calories 86, Fat calories 9, Fat 1 g, Saturated fat 0 g, Cholesterol 0 mg, Protein 3 g, Carbohydrate 20 g, Dietary fiber 3 g, Sodium 5 mg, Calories from fat 10%, Calories from saturated fat 0%

**Allowances:** ⅛ fat + 1 starch + ⅛ vegetable

# STEWED POTATOES, GREEN BEANS, AND ZUCCHINI

This lovely vegetable dish is a meal unto itself, very satisfying and filling.

1 teaspoon extra virgin olive oil
1 cup onion, chopped
2 baking potatoes, large, peeled and cubed
1 cup zucchini, cubed
2 cups green beans, cut in half
3 cups tomato, freshly diced
½ teaspoon dried oregano
¼ cup parsley, freshly chopped
¼ cup dill
1 tablespoon lemon juice
¼ teaspoon black pepper, freshly ground

In a large pot, heat olive oil on medium heat, then sauté onion. Stir in potatoes and ¾ cup water. Increase heat until the mixture simmers lightly. Cover and cook about 10 minutes or until potatoes are tender. Add more water if necessary. Stir in zucchini, green beans, tomatoes, oregano, and ½ to ¾ cup water. Return to a simmer, cover, and cook about 10 minutes or until veggies are tender. Stir in parsley, dill, lemon juice, and pepper.

YIELD: 8 servings (½ cup per serving)

**Each serving contains approximately:** Calories 107, Fat calories 18, Fat 2 g, Saturated fat 0 g, Cholesterol 0 mg, Protein 4 g, Carbohydrate 22 g, Dietary fiber 5 g, Sodium 19 mg, Calories from fat 17%, Calories from saturated fat 0%

**Allowances:** ⅛ fat + 1 starch + ⅞ vegetable

# ROASTED ARTICHOKES ALLA ROSATI

These are so good and so easy, we agreed they are a "basic," a "must always have on hand" item. If you like artichokes, they make virtually everything taste better with their addition: from salads to bruschetta to risotto, they simply take a good dish to incredible in seconds. Having them always readily available inspires dishes like Chess' Roasted Artichoke Salad (page 210), made by my eight-year-old, Chess.

2 9-ounce packages of Bird's Eye frozen Deluxe Artichoke Hearts
I tablespoon extra virgin olive oil
Freshly ground black pepper

Defrost artichoke hearts and toss with olive oil. Place under the broiler and cook about 15 minutes, turning once. They are ready when they look slightly browned or roasted on both sides. Remove from the oven and top with freshly ground black pepper. You can marinate them in the fridge and enjoy as a topping for days.

VARIATION: Unless you are adding them to a dish already flavorful, you may want to add balsamic vinegar or freshly squeezed lemon or lime juice for a nice punch.

NOTE: The only way to make them better is when the fresh baby artichokes are available in the produce market. When you have time during the artichoke season, try My Favorite Thistle, the Artichoke in my previous book, *Heal Your Heart*.

YIELD: Makes 6 servings of about 12 artichokes each

**Each serving contains approximately:** Calories 34, Fat calories 22, Fat 2.5 g, Saturated fat 0, Cholesterol 0, Protein .7 g, Carbohydrate 2.3 g, Dietary fiber 1.7 g, Sodium 18, Calories from fat 65%, Calories from saturated fat 0%

**Allowances:** ½ fat + ½ vegetable

# STUFFED ARTICHOKES

This is another great way to enjoy artichokes. The stuffing is filling so this can be a stand-alone meal, especially with a side of beans.

4 fresh artichokes
2 Toufayan Salt Free Pitas, diced
6 grape tomatoes, diced
I cup yellow onion, diced
I tablespoon garlic, minced
I teaspoon fresh basil
I teaspoon black pepper
I teaspoon honey
½ cup tomato puree, no-salt added

Preheat oven to 350 degrees F. Trim about one-third off the top of each artichoke, remove the light colored center leaves—not the heart—and place in a small pan. Combine ¼ cup water and remaining ingredients (except tomato puree) in a pan and sauté until onions are lightly browned. Add a little more water if the mixture is too dry. Use this mixture to stuff the middle of each artichoke. Mix tomato puree and ¾ cup water in a small bowl. Pour mixture into pan—it should fill up no more than half the pan. Cover and bake for 1 hour. Uncover and bake for 15 to 20 minutes. Plate artichokes and top with liquid from pan.

YIELD: 4 servings

**Each serving contains approximately:** Calories 155, Fat calories 5, Fat 0.5 g, Saturated fat 0 g, Cholesterol 0 mg, Protein 13 g, Carbohydrate 59 g, Dietary fiber 10 g, Sodium 137 mg, Calories from fat 3%, Calories from saturated fat 0%

**Allowances:** ¼ starch + 5 vegetables

# SWEET AND SOUR ONIONS

These onions will melt in your mouth!

3 red onions, halved and thinly sliced
1 tablespoon extra virgin olive oil
2 garlic cloves, thinly sliced
⅛ teaspoon red pepper flakes
½ cup *Vegetable Stock*, no salt added
1 tablespoon parsley leaves, freshly chopped
6 tablespoons balsamic vinegar
1 tablespoon honey

Parboil the sliced onion for about 2 to 3 minutes. Drain well and set aside.

Heat the oil and add the garlic and red pepper flakes for about 5 minutes. Add the onions, vegetable stock, and parsley leaves, stir well and bring to a boil. Reduce the heat to low, and simmer for about 10 minutes. Add vinegar and honey and cook for 2 to 3 minutes.

YIELD: 4 servings

**Each serving contains approximately:** Calories 83, Fat calories 23, Fat 3 g, Saturated fat 0.5 g, Cholesterol 0 mg, Protein 1 g, Carbohydrate 15 g, Dietary fiber 1 g, Sodium 11 mg, Calories from fat 28%, Calories from saturated fat 5%

**Allowances:** ¾ fat + ⅓ starch + 1 vegetable

# SWISS CHARD

For most, Swiss chard is an acquired taste. Our chef, J.R., pairs this dish with sweet potato pie, and many love it with any potato dish.

I teaspoon extra virgin olive oil
I tablespoon garlic, minced
6 cups Swiss chard, chopped
I teaspoon honey

Sauté garlic in oil about one minute. Add ½ cup water, then the Swiss chard. Cover for 2 to 3 minutes, stir well, add another ½ cup of water and honey, stir well, and cover again. Cook 3 to 4 minutes, then remove from heat, mix well again, cover, and let sit for 2 to 3 minutes.

NOTE: If the dish is too bitter for your taste, add a little more honey.

YIELD: 2 servings (¾ cup per serving)

**Each serving contains approximately:** Calories 62, Fat calories 18, Fat 2 g, Saturated fat 0.3 g, Cholesterol 0 mg, Protein 2 g, Carbohydrate 10 g, Dietary fiber 2 g, Sodium 161 mg, Calories from fat 29%, Calories from saturated fat 4%

**Allowances:** ½ fat + 2 vegetables

# COASTAL PICKLED RED CABBAGE

The following recipe just goes to show you that it's possible to eat something delicious even where others are choosing everything fried! Herron's Family Restaurant in Duck, North Carolina, has been owned and operated since 1985, and looks like a dieter's nightmare until you get creative with the menu—and the owner, Mike Campbell. I befriended Mike, who was kind enough to steer me to their pickled red cabbage, and then actually gave me the recipe! Although I modified the recipe by halving the sugar, you can also use apple juice concentrate instead to make it more nutrient dense.

¾ teaspoon extra virgin olive oil
½ head red cabbage, julienned
1½ cups red wine vinegar
6 tablespoons brown sugar

Heat olive oil and sauté red cabbage for 5 to 10 minutes. Add the remaining ingredients and refrigerate. This is very good within an hour, but even better the next day.

YIELD: 8 servings

**Each serving contains approximately:** Calories 54, Fat calories 5, Fat 0.5 g, Saturated fat 0 g, Cholesterol 0 g, Protein 1 g, Carbohydrate 13 g, Dietary fiber 1 g, Sodium 14 mg, Calories from fat 9%, Calories from saturated fat 0%

**Allowances:** ⅒ fat + ⅓ fruit + 1 vegetable

# ORANGE RICE

This rice recipe hails from New England. It's both tasty and easy to make and blends with most chicken and fish dishes.

1 cup brown rice
1 cup orange juice
½ cup raisins, or more if desired
2 tablespoons orange zest, finely chopped

Toast uncooked brown rice over medium heat about 4 minutes, stirring often—do not let rice burn. Add 1 cup water, orange juice, and raisins, cover, reduce to low heat, and simmer 30 to 45 minutes or until liquid is absorbed and rice is tender. Stir occasionally. Add orange zest, stir, and cook an additional 5 minutes.

Yield: 10 servings (⅓ cup per serving)

**Each serving contains approximately:** Calories 107, Fat calories 5.4, Fat 0.6 g, Saturated fat 0 g, Cholesterol 0 mg, Protein 2 g, Carbohydrate 23 g, Dietary fiber 1.2 g, Sodium 4 mg, Calories from fat 5%, Calories from saturated fat 0%

**Allowances:** ⅛ starch + ⅜ fruit

# RACHELLE'S MEXICAN BAKED BEANS

This recipe is adapted from *Beyond the Moon*, a cookbook by Ginny Callahan (HarperCollins, 1996). This dish requires very little preparation and has lots of flavor!

1 tablespoon canola oil

2 cups red onion, chopped

6 garlic cloves, minced

4 raw jalapeño peppers, minced

2 cups red bell peppers, chopped

1 tablespoon cumin

1¼ cups tomato sauce, no salt added

1 tablespoon honey

1 tablespoon molasses

2 tablespoons Dijon mustard, no salt added

1 15-ounce can pinto beans (Eden)

1 15-ounce can Great Northern beans (Eden)

Preheat the oven to 350 degrees F.

Heat a heavy pan or deep skillet and add oil. Sauté onions for a few minutes—to your liking. Add garlic, jalapeños, bell pepper, and cumin and sauté for a few more minutes. Stir in the tomato sauce, honey, molasses, mustard, and all the beans. Reseason as needed with cumin and pepper.

Pour this mixture into an oven-safe dish and bake, uncovered, for at least 30 minutes. The longer you cook it, the more the beans will "set up" as the liquid is driven into the beans and to the atmosphere.

YIELD: 6 servings (1 cup per serving)

**Each serving contains approximately:** Calories 224, Fat calories 32, Fat 3.5 g, Saturated fat 0 g, Cholesterol 0 mg, Protein 9 g, Carbohydrate 42 g, Dietary fiber 11 g, Sodium 79 mg, Calories from fat 14%, Calories from saturated fat 0%

**Allowances:** ½ fat + 2 starches + 1½ vegetables

# SOUPS

These homemade soups are delicious and a refreshing alternative to the salt-laden soups found in cans or at restaurants.

## BOUILLABAISSE

This is traditionally served at the Rice House for Christmas dinner. It is one of our top 5 favorite meals. Buon Natale! Buon giorno! Salud!

2 tablespoons extra virgin olive oil
¼ cup onions, finely chopped
4 leeks, finely julienned (white portion only)
4 tomatoes, medium-size, skinned, pulp squeezed out, and diced
5 garlic cloves
1 tablespoon fresh fennel, finely chopped
½–1 teaspoon saffron spice
2 tablespoons bay leaves, pulverized
2 tablespoons tomato paste, no salt added
½ teaspoon celery seed
3 tablespoons parsley, freshly chopped
1 tablespoon black pepper, freshly ground
1 lobster, cut into 1-inch pieces
12 clams, medium
12 mussels, medium
12 shrimp, medium
1 pound snapper fillet, cut into 2-inch pieces
1 pound Atlantic/Pacific halibut fillet, cut into 2-inch pieces
2½ cups hot fish stock, no salt added

Prepare above ingredients. In a large pot, heat 2 tablespoons of olive oil. When the oil is hot, add the vegetable ingredients and cook until they are transparent. You may prefer to leave the fish in 2-inch-thick slices and use some smaller fish whole. If so, add the thinner pieces or small scrubbed shellfish to the pot slightly later than the thicker ones, but do not disturb the boiling. Cover with the fish stock. Keep the heat high and force the boiling, which should continue for 15 to 20 minutes.

YIELD: 10 servings

**Each serving contains approximately:** Calories 239, Fat calories 76, Fat 8.4 g, Saturated fat 1 g, Cholesterol 68 mg, Protein 30 g, Carbohydrate 11 g, Dietary fiber 2 g, Sodium 205 mg, Omega-3 0.5 g, Calories from fat 32%, Calories from saturated fat 4%

**Allowances:** ⅜ fat + 4 proteins + ½ vegetable

# MINESTRONE ALLA ROSATI

This recipe for minestrone absolutely must be made with savoy cabbage. We've tried other cabbages, but the taste is just not the same.

1 tablespoon extra virgin olive oil
4 anchovies, chopped
2 carrots, chopped
2 onions, chopped
9 garlic cloves, sliced
¼ cup parsley, chopped
2 tablespoons rosemary, chopped
1 bunch kale, cleaned and shredded
1 Savoy cabbage head, thinly sliced
2 28-ounce cans Italian tomatoes, no salt added, put through food
    mill (or coarsely chopped)
Parmigiano rind

Black pepper, to taste
2 15-ounce cans cannellini beans, no salt added

Heat olive oil over medium heat. Add chopped anchovies, carrots, onions, garlic, parsley, and rosemary, and cook about 7 minutes. Add kale and when cooked down add cabbage. Cook until cabbage softens, about 5 minutes. Add tomatoes and Parmigiano rind. Season with black pepper. Cook 10 minutes, stirring several times.

Rinse cannellini beans under cold water. Smash the beans from one can with potato masher and add along with can of whole beans to minestrone. Simmer 20 minutes longer over low heat.

YIELD: 6 servings

**Each serving contains approximately:** Calories 213, Fat calories 34, Fat 3.8 g, Saturated fat 0.6 g, Cholesterol 2 mg, Protein 10 g, Carbohydrate 38 g, Dietary fiber 9 g, Sodium 254 mg, Calories from fat 16%, Calories from saturated fat 3%

**Allowances:** ½ fat + 1 starch + ¹⁄₁₀ protein + 4 vegetables


# SPLIT PEA SOUP

This Rice House favorite surprises everyone because it is so rich in taste without the traditional ham hock to flavor it.

4 cups *Vegetable Stock* (page 198), or canned, no-salt-added vegetable
    stock (Perfect Addition)
1¼ cups split peas
1¼ carrots, chopped
¾ cup yellow onion, chopped
1 teaspoon thyme
1 teaspoon basil
1 teaspoon black pepper
2 bay leaves

Boil peas in stock for 1 hour, stirring occasionally. Reduce heat to low-medium, add all other ingredients, cover, and cook 45 to 55 more minutes, stirring occasionally. Remove bay leaves before serving.

YIELD: 15 servings

**Each serving contains approximately:** Calories 69, Fat calories 7, Fat 0.8 g, Saturated fat 0 g, Cholesterol 0 mg, Protein 5 g, Carbohydrate 12 g, Dietary fiber 5 g, Sodium 45 mg, Calories from fat 10%, Calories from saturated fat 0%

**Allowances:** ¾ starch + ¼ vegetable

# RACHELLE'S CREAMY CARROT SOUP WITH MINT

Adapted from a recipe by Chef Albert H. Chase, Jr., Institute for Culinary Awakening, made without added sodium. This delicious soup thrives on the subtle contrast between the sweet carrots and the mint. It's both refreshing and filling.

2 tablespoons canola oil
2 cups onions, diced
4 cups carrots, diced
4 garlic cloves, sliced
Pinch of cayenne pepper
2 cups *Vegetable Stock* (page 198)
¼ cup parsley, chopped
2 tablespoons fresh mint
½ cup rolled oats

Heat a heavy-bottomed soup pot for 1 minute, then add the oil; heat for an additional minute. Add onions and sauté for 5 minutes until soft, then add carrots and cook for another 5 minutes. Add garlic and pepper and cook for about 2 minutes. Add 4 cups water and *Veg-*

*etable Stock* and bring to a boil. Reduce heat and simmer for about 30 minutes. Add the parsley, mint, and oats and cook for 10 minutes (you can also use cooked rice or potato instead of the oats). Remove the pot from the heat and cool for about 10 minutes on a cooling rack. Puree the mixture until smooth. Reheat for serving or refrigerate. The soup can be served cold or hot.

YIELD: 8 servings (1 cup per serving)

**Each serving contains approximately:** Calories 110, Fat calories 45, Fat 5 g, Saturated fat 0 g, Cholesterol 0 mg, Protein 3 g, Carbohydrate 15 g, Dietary fiber 4 g, Sodium 80 mg, Calories from fat 41%, Calories from saturated fat 0%

**Allowances:** ¾ fat + ⅓ starch + 2 vegetables

# RACHELLE'S CURRIED LENTIL SOUP WITH MANGO

This dish was born out of a random list of ingredients provided to Rachelle by the participants. Modeled after a recipe from Diane Shaw's *Almost Vegetarian Entertaining* (Three Rivers, 1998), this makes a wonderfully flavorful and hearty vegetarian entrée but can also be served in a smaller portion as a fantastic first course. There are numerous variations on a theme with this dish. Exercise your own preferences by adjusting either the type of lentils used (green versus red), the amount of each seasoning/spice used, adding or deleting specific spices, and by substituting another fruit for the mango.

1 cup lentils, red (pink), uncooked
1 Yukon Gold potato, medium
1½ teaspoons olive oil
1 red onion, medium, chopped
1 red bell pepper, large, chopped

2 teaspoons cumin

I teaspoon coriander

½ teaspoon turmeric

¼ teaspoon cayenne pepper

2 tablespoons fresh ginger, grated

¼ cup tomato paste, no salt added

I fresh mango, medium, chopped

2 tablespoons fresh cilantro, minced

Place the lentils in a saucepan and cover with about 3 inches of water. Bring to a simmer and cover. Cook the lentils until tender, about 20 minutes.

Wash the potato, pierce, and cook in the microwave for about 4 minutes or until done. When cool enough to handle, cut into cubes.

Add oil to heated skillet and sauté onion for about 3 to 5 minutes over medium heat. Add bell pepper and all the herbs and spices (except for the cilantro) to the skillet and continue to sauté for a few more minutes. Mix in tomato paste and then remove from heat.

Using an immersion wand (or a blender or food processor), puree the lentils in their cooking liquid until smooth. Add mango and potato to the lentils and puree again until smooth. Add the contents of the skillet to the saucepan and stir in well. Recheck your seasonings here and make adjustments as necessary to meet your preferences. Stir in minced cilantro and serve hot.

YIELD: 4 servings (1½ cups per serving)

**Each serving contains approximately:** Calories 338, Fat calories 36, Fat 4 g, Saturated fat 0.5 g, Cholesterol 0 mg, Protein 15 g, Carbohydrate 64 g, Dietary fiber 10 g, Sodium 30 mg, Calories from fat 11%, Calories from saturated fat 1%

**Allowances:** ⅜ fat + 3 starches + 2 vegetables + ½ fruit

# GAZPACHO

This gazpacho is as refreshing as it is flavorful, with just the right amount of kick.

I cucumber, large, cubed
10 tomatoes, ripe, seeded and cubed
I green pepper, chopped
I yellow pepper, chopped
I Vidalia onion, diced
2 garlic gloves, sliced
½ lemon, peeled and seeded
½ tablespoon wine vinegar, red or white
6 pitas, no salt added, diced
4 drops hot sauce
2 tablespoons olive oil
Pepper, to taste
Honey (optional), to taste
I stalk celery

You can make this soup entirely in the food processor. Simply blend the diced bread with all the other ingredients. Add a few ice cubes. Chill for 1 hour. Pour a 6-ounce serving in a bowl and garnish with snipped young celery leaves. Add pepper to taste. Enjoy!

YIELD: 6 servings (6 ounces per serving)

**Each serving contains approximately:** Calories 142, Fat calories 45, Fat 5 g, Saturated fat 0.7 g, Cholesterol 0 mg, Protein 6 g, Carbohydrate 33 g, Dietary fiber 4 g, Sodium 29 mg, Calories from fat 32%, Calories from saturated fat 4%

**Allowances:** 1 fat + ⅜ starch + 2¾ vegetables

# ENTREES

These main dishes are all-star attractions—on their own or paired with vegetables, salad, or dessert.

## J.R.'S CRABFREE CRAB CAKES

Absolutely everyone will think it's crab! This is a seafood favorite at the Rice House.

½ teaspoon olive oil

12 ounce sea bass fillet, raw

3 ounces fresh lemon juice

1 onion, raw, chopped

1½ cups organic tomato puree, no added salt

¼ teaspoon black pepper

2 teaspoons fresh basil, chopped

3 fresh garlic cloves

½ teaspoon extra virgin olive oil

3 whole wheat pita pocket breads, 6½ inches, chopped

⅛ cup sweet red bell pepper, chopped

⅛ cup sweet green bell pepper, chopped

Coat a 13 x 9–inch baking pan with olive oil. Place the fish in the pan, add 3 ounces water and lemon juice and bake at 350 degrees F for 7 to 10 minutes. Set aside.

Place remaining ingredients in a large mixing bowl and mix well. Set aside.

Carefully remove fish from pan and dice. Add fish to dry ingredients and mix well. If the mixture is too dry, add fish juice from the baking pan to moisten.

Coat a large cookie sheet with olive oil. Form mixture into 6 patties and place them onto the cookie sheet. Bake at 350 degrees F until crispy and slightly brown, approximately 10 minutes.

YIELD: 6 servings

**Each serving contains approximately:** Calories 182, Fat calories 23, Fat 3 g, Saturated fat 0.5 g, Cholesterol 23 mg, Protein 15 g, Carbohydrate 27 g, Dietary fiber 5 g, Omega-3 38g, Sodium 232 mg (103 mg if pita is low-sodium), Calories from fat 2%, Calories from saturated fat 15%

**Allowances:** 2 proteins + ½ starch + 1¼ vegetables

# J.R.'S LASAGNA

Mama never made it so good! This lasagne is hearty, chewy, and healthy.

1 teaspoon extra virgin olive oil
2 cups yellow onion, diced
1 tablespoon minced garlic
1 teaspoon fresh basil, chopped
1 teaspoon fresh oregano
1 teaspoon cayenne pepper
1 cup textured soy protein (TVP)
6 cherry tomatoes, diced
3 cups cauliflower, boiled then pureed
3 cups spinach
1½ cups Basic Tomato Sauce, page 193
10 lasagne noodles

Preheat oven to 350 degrees F. Heat olive oil in a large pan over low heat and then add onions, garlic, and spices; sauté until lightly browned. Add TVP, cherry tomatoes, and cauliflower puree mixed with spinach and ¾ cup of Basic Tomato Sauce. Coat a small 8 x 8–inch pan with a little olive oil, lay lasagne noodles across the bottom—you may have to break the noodles. Spread approximately ¼ of the mixture on top of the lasagne noodles, alternating noodles and mixture for 4 layers. Cover with foil and cook 35 minutes. Plate and spoon a little tomato sauce over each, then serve.

YIELD: 8 servings

**Each serving contains approximately:** Calories 243, Fat calories 18, Fat 2 g, Saturated fat 0 g, Cholesterol 0 mg, Protein 22 g, Carbohydrate 38 g, Dietary fiber 5 g, Omega-3 38g, Sodium 22 mg, Calories from fat 7%, Calories from saturated fat 0%

**Allowances:** ⅛ fat + 1⅓ protein + 1½ starches + 1¾ vegetables

# RICE HOUSE MEATLOAF

A Rice House favorite, this meatloaf dish stands alone: it's flavorful, hearty, and we doubt you'll have room for dessert!

2 cups textured soy protein (TVP)
I teaspoon extra virgin olive oil
1½ cups sweet onion, diced
I red bell pepper, diced
I yellow bell pepper, diced
I green bell pepper, diced
I tablespoon garlic, minced
¼ cup balsamic vinegar
I pinch black pepper
I pinch cayenne pepper
I pinch oregano
I pinch fresh basil
¼ cup tomato puree, no salt added
I teaspoon honey, optional
3 Toufayan Salt Free Pitas, diced

Preheat oven to 350 degrees F. Set TVP in a strainer, pour 3 cups boiling water over it, let drain, and set aside. In a pot, heat olive oil on medium heat. Add onions, bell peppers, and garlic; sauté until lightly browned. Add balsamic vinegar and spices and sauté for 2 to 3 minutes. Add TVP, tomato puree, and honey and stir well. Cover and leave on low heat for 2 to 3 minutes, stirring often. Add diced pita bread and mix well. Remove from heat, but leave pot covered for 2 to 3 minutes. Coat a meatloaf pan lightly with olive oil, pour in mixture, and bake for 30 to 40 minutes.

YIELD: 12 servings

**Each serving contains approximately:** Calories 171, Fat calories 9, Fat 1 g, Saturated fat 0 g, Cholesterol 0 mg, Protein 33 g, Carbohydrate 25 g, Dietary fiber 3 g, Sodium 5 mg, Calories from fat 5%, Calories from saturated fat 0%

**Allowances:** ¹⁄₁₂ fat + 2½ proteins + ⅛ starch + ½ vegetable

# KYM'S TANDOORI CHICKEN

Tandoori is a method of cooking using a clay oven with a coal or wood fire. Popular in Pakistan and India, tandoori cooking is gaining popularity in Europe and the United States. But, this recipe has been successfully prepared in a porcelain Dutch oven!

1 3-pound chicken
¼ teaspoon dry mustard
1 cup plain nonfat organic yogurt
¼ cup lemon juice
3 garlic cloves, chopped
½ teaspoon ground cardamom
¼ teaspoon ground ginger
¼ teaspoon ground cumin
¼ teaspoon crushed red pepper
¼ teaspoon black pepper

Wash chicken, remove skin, and place in a large glass bowl. Combine ½ teaspoon water and dry mustard to create a paste, add yogurt, lemon juice, garlic, cardamom, ginger, cumin, red pepper, and black pepper. Pour over the chicken to coat well. Cover bowl with plastic wrap and place in refrigerator.

Preheat the oven to 375 degrees F. Remove chicken from bowl and transfer to rack in shallow roasting pan. Reserve marinade to use for basting during roasting. Roast uncovered at 375 degrees F for approximately 2 hours. Spoon reserved marinade over chicken during the last 30 minutes of roasting time. Place foil over chicken parts that are roasting faster than breast area.

Remove chicken from pan, then slice and serve.

YIELD: 12 servings

**Each serving contains approximately:** Calories 213, Fat calories 69, Fat 7.7 g, Saturated Fat 2.1 g, Cholesterol 95 mg, Protein 32 g, Carbohydrates 2.4 g, Dietary fiber 0.1 g, Sodium 91 mg, Calories from fat 33%, Calories from saturated fat 9%

**Allowances:** 3 proteins + 1½ vegetables + ¼ fruit

# CARIBBEAN CHICKEN WITH LIMES

The food of the Caribbean is very international, reflecting the influences of the many countries that founded the islands. This recipe, donated by Kym Stork, incorporates flavors from Britain (Worcestershire sauce and lime), Spain (cabbage and onion), and Mexico (tomatoes).

1 2-pound chicken, cut up, without skin
4 tablespoons fresh lime juice
1 tablespoon extra virgin olive oil
2 tomatoes, chopped

1 sweet onion, chopped

1 celery stalk, chopped

3 garlic cloves, chopped

2 teaspoons Worcestershire sauce, low-sodium

⅛ teaspoon pepper

1 cup brown rice, uncooked

1 tablespoon parsley, chopped

2 teaspoons vegetarian bouillon, dry

½ teaspoon grated lime peel

4 cups cabbage, shredded

Place chicken in shallow glass or plastic dish. Pour lime juice over chicken. Cover and refrigerate for approximately 1 hour. Heat olive oil in Dutch oven until hot. Cook chicken over medium heat for approximately 15 minutes.

Drain fat from Dutch oven, then add ¼ cup water, chopped vegetables, Worcestershire sauce, and pepper. Heat to boiling; reduce heat, cover, and simmer for 30 minutes.

Heat 2 cups water, rice, parsley, bouillon, and lime peel to a boil, stirring once or twice. Reduce heat; simmer for about 45 minutes.

Add cabbage to Dutch oven. Cover and simmer for another 10 to 15 minutes.

Lightly fluff rice with a fork; cover and let steam while Dutch oven is simmering.

Remove chicken from Dutch oven and shred. Add shredded chicken back into Dutch oven and stir.

Using a fork, layer rice into the bottom of a casserole pan. Cover rice with shredded chicken mixture, including juice. Serve hot.

YIELD: 8 servings

**Each serving contains approximately:** Calories 318, Fat calories 91, Fat 10 g, Saturated fat 2.4 g, Cholesterol 94 g, Protein 34 g, Carbohydrates 23 g, Dietary fiber 2.3 g, Sodium 116 mg, Calories from fat 28%, Calories from saturated fat 7%

**Allowances:** ⅓ fat + 3 proteins + 1 starch + 2 vegetables

# RISOTTO WITH GRILLED SWORDFISH

This is one of Bob's signature dishes. The participants have been begging for this recipe for years.

BASIC RISOTTO

6 cups *Vegetable Stock* (p. 198) (or no-salt-added vegetable stock)
2 tablespoons extra virgin olive oil
1 onion, medium (I prefer organic red), chopped
2 cups arborio rice
1 cup dry white wine
¼ cup parsley, chopped (to be added after sauce, see below)
Red pepper flakes, to taste

¾ pound swordfish, grilled and cut into small pieces or mashed

Heat the stock.

Heat the olive oil in a large saucepan over medium heat. Add the chopped onion and cook, stirring, until the onion is soft. Add the rice, stir, and cook 3 minutes. Add the wine and cook until the wine is almost gone. Add stock to just cover the rice and cook, stirring, until the stock is almost completely absorbed. Continue adding stock, stirring and cooking in this manner until the rice is tender.

Stir the swordfish into the rice and cook for 1 to 2 minutes. Add parsley and red pepper flakes and serve.

YIELD: 6 servings

**Each serving contains approximately:** Calories 274, Fat calories 77, Fat 8.6 g, Saturated fat 1.5 g, Cholesterol 28 mg, Protein 22 g, Carbohydrate 26 g, Dietary Fiber 1 g, Sodium 134 mg, Omega-3 0.6 g, Calories from fat 27%, Calories from saturated fat 5%

**Allowances:** 1 fat + 1⅗ proteins + 1⅗ starches + ⅙ vegetable

# RISOTTO WITH GRILLED VEGETABLES

Grilled vegetables give this risotto dish a lot of color, texture, and varied flavors, as well as being packed with antioxidants.

BASIC RISOTTO

6 cups *Vegetable Stock* (p. 196) (or no-salt-added vegetable stock)
2 tablespoons extra virgin olive oil
1 onion, medium (I prefer organic red), chopped
2 cups arborio rice
1 cup dry white wine
¼ cup parsley, chopped (to be added after sauce; see below)

GRILLED VEGETABLES

4 carrots, medium, halved and cut into quarters lengthwise
2 onions, medium, quartered
2 red bell peppers, cored and cleaned
1 tablespoon extra virgin olive oil
½ cup Parmigiano Reggiano cheese (heart patients may prefer
    to omit)

Prepare as for Risotto with Grilled Swordfish (p. 263).

YIELD: 6 servings

**Each serving contains approximately:** Calories 260, Fat calories 75, Fat 8.3 g, Saturated fat 1 g, Cholesterol 0 mg, Protein 4 g, Carbohydrate 36 g, Dietary fiber 3 g, Sodium 99 mg, Calories from fat 28%, Calories from saturated fat 3%

**Allowances:** 1½ fats, 1⅗ starches; 1½ vegetables, ½ protein.

# VEGETARIAN RAGU

Another great use for TVP, this Italian-style dish packs a wallop of flavor and nutrition. It's also easy and quick to make in either small servings or for a big group.

2 teaspoons extra virgin olive oil

2 onions, medium, chopped in large dice

6 garlic cloves, thinly sliced

2 tablespoons fennel seeds

Pinch red pepper flakes

1 pound TVP (texturized vegetable protein)

1 tablespoon tomato paste, no salt added

2 28-ounce cans peeled whole tomatoes, no salt added, crushed by hand

1 cup red wine

½ cup nonfat ricotta cheese or cottage cheese (nonfat, no salt added)

2 tablespoons parsley leaves, chopped

Freshly ground black pepper

1 pound rigatoni pasta

¼ cup fennel fronds, chopped

¼ cup Parmesan cheese, grated

In a 3-quart saucepan, make the vegetarian ragu by heating 1 teaspoon olive oil over medium heat. Add the onion and cook until soft and light golden brown, about 7 to 8 minutes. Add the garlic, fennel seeds, and pepper flakes and stir to combine. Add the TVP, the tomato paste, canned tomatoes, and red wine. Bring the sauce to a boil. Lower the heat and let the sauce simmer for about 30 minutes before removing the pan from the heat.

In a bowl, combine the ricotta with 1 teaspoon olive oil, chopped parsley, and black pepper. Set aside.

Bring 6 quarts of water to a boil. Cook the rigatoni according to the directions on the package. Drain. Toss the cooked noodles in the vegetarian ragu with the ricotta mixture and fennel fronds, and garnish with Parmesan.

YIELD: 15 servings

**Each serving contains approximately:** Calories 260, Fat calories 23, Fat 2.6 g, Saturated fat 0.5 g, Cholesterol 4 mg, Protein 25 g, Carbohydrate 38 g, Dietary fiber 7 g, Sodium 137 mg, Calories from fat 9%, Calories from saturated fat 2%

**Allowances:** ⅛ fat + 1½ proteins + 1½ starches + 2 vegetables

# LENTIL DAL WITH FRESH GINGER, GREEN CHILIES, AND CILANTRO

This recipe is adapted from *Indian Home Cooking* by Suvir Saran and Stephanie Lyness (Clarkson Potter Publishers, 2004). For those of you who like Indian spices, you will simply delight in this subtle yet tangy dish.

LENTILS

I cup lentils, pink, uncooked
½ teaspoon turmeric

TEMPERING OIL

I½ tablespoons canola oil
I¼ teaspoons cumin seeds
I–2 red chilies, dried, whole
I tablespoon fresh ginger, minced
I teaspoon garlic, minced
I green chili, hot, minced
½ teaspoon cayenne pepper

¼–½ cup cilantro, freshly chopped

Juice from ½ lemon or lime

3 cups cooked basmati rice

Pick over the lentils, wash, and drain.

Place lentils into a saucepan with 2 to 3 cups water and turmeric and bring to a boil.

Skim well, reduce heat, and simmer, covered, until lentils are soft, approximately 15 to 20 minutes. Add additional water as needed to keep lentils moist. Mash some of the lentils with a spoon to make them thicker or add water to make them thinner, as you prefer. Simmer, uncovered, for 5 more minutes to thicken.

For the tempering oil: place the oil and the cumin seeds in a small frying pan over medium-high heat. Cook until cumin turns a light brown, about 1 to 2 minutes. Add the dried chilies, ginger, garlic, and green chili and cook until garlic turns golden brown, about 30 more seconds. Remove pan from heat and add cayenne and add a few drops of water to stop the cooking (but watch for possible splatter). Stir the tempering oil, half of the cilantro, and all the lemon/lime juice into the *dal* and simmer gently for 5 minutes. Transfer the *dal* (pink lentils) to a serving bowl and sprinkle with remaining cilantro. Serve hot over steaming basmati rice.

YIELD: 4 servings (¾ cup cooked rice per serving)

**Each serving contains approximately:** Calories 380, Fat calories 63, Fat 7 g, Saturated Fat 0.6 g, Cholesterol 0 mg, Protein 16 g, Carbohydrate 63 g, Dietary fiber 7 g, Sodium 8 mg, Calories from fat 17%, Calories from saturated fat 1%

**Allowances:** 1⅛ fat + 4 starches + ¼ vegetable

# RACHELLE'S NORTH AFRICAN COUSCOUS PAELLA

This recipe is adapted from *Moosewood Restaurant Cooks at Home*, The Moosewood Collective (Simon & Schuster, 1994), made without added sodium or butter. Another dish that delivers subtle yet interesting flavors. Once you've tried it with shrimp, try it with monkfish.

1½ tablespoons olive oil
1 cup red bell pepper, chopped
1 cup scallions, chopped
4 garlic cloves, minced
2 teaspoons coriander
1 teaspoon turmeric
Black pepper to taste
Pinch of cayenne pepper
4 cups *Vegetable Stock* (p. 198) or Perfect Addition bouillon
½ block tofu (Nasoya brand), firm style, cut into cubes
½ pound shrimp
2 cups green beans, frozen
2 cups couscous, dry
2 teaspoons toasted sesame oil
Lemon to taste

Heat a heavy-bottomed soup pot for 1 minute and then add the oil; heat for an additional minute. Add the peppers, scallions, garlic, coriander, turmeric, and black and cayenne peppers and sauté on medium heat for 3 to 4 minutes. Stir in the *Vegetable Stock*. Add the tofu and shrimp (cleaned and deveined) and cook for another 3 to 4 minutes until the tofu is hot and shrimp are pink. Stir in the green beans and cook for 1 more minute. Stir in the couscous and the sesame oil. Cover and remove from the heat. Leave the lid on. Let stand for at least 5 minutes so that the couscous will take up the broth. Uncover the pot and topple out gently into a serving dish, being sure to break up any clumps. You have a beautiful and healthy main course to serve your guests or lunch to take to work for several days. Enjoy!

YIELD: 10 servings (1 cup per serving)

**Each serving contains approximately:** Calories 227, Fat calories 45, Fat 5 g, Saturated fat 0.5 g, Cholesterol 59 mg, Protein 13 g, Carbohydrate 32 g, Dietary fiber 3 g, Omega-3s 0.12 g, Sodium 93 mg, Calories from fat 20%, Calories from saturated fat 2%

**Allowances:** ⅔ fat + 1 protein + 1⅔ starches + ⅔ vegetable

You can substitute any frozen vegetable for the green beans, e.g. peas, and then adjust your numbers.

# RACHELLE'S "TWO STEW"

This is an easy dish to make that's healthful and hearty with a little edge. Makes plenty for leftovers, for lunches, or to freeze.

1 tablespoon canola oil
1 cup yellow onion, medium, chopped
4 garlic cloves, minced
2 teaspoons cumin
2 teaspoons coriander
2 teaspoons tarragon
¼ teaspoon paprika
¼ teaspoon cayenne
Freshly ground black pepper, to taste
1 15-ounce can diced tomatoes (DelMonte), no salt added
1 15-ounce can aduki beans (Eden)
1 15-ounce can black beans (Eden)
1 15-ounce can canned corn (DelMonte), no salt added
2 cups white rice, cooked

Heat a heavy pan or deep skillet and add oil. Sauté onions for a few minutes—to your liking. Add garlic and spices and sauté for a few more minutes. Stir in all the tomatoes, beans, corn, and rice. Stir in 2 cups water. Reseason as needed with cumin, pepper, and so on. Let simmer for at least 15 minutes to allow seasonings to mingle.

YIELD: 8 servings (1 cup per serving)

**Each serving contains approximately:** Calories 218, Fat calories 22, Fat 2.4 g, Saturated fat 0 g, Cholesterol 0 mg, Protein 9 g, Carbohydrate 42 g, Dietary fiber 8 g, Sodium 36 mg, Calories from fat 10%, Calories from saturated fat 0%

**Allowances:** ⅜ fat + 2¼ starches + ⅔ vegetable

# RACHELLE'S MARINATED TOFU CUTLETS

Tofu is an enigma for most of us, often leading us to ask ourselves, "What to do with tofu?" Tofu is made from soybeans and is a wonderful source of protein and calcium. It does pack a few calories, though, so keep an eye on the portions. Here then is tofu, boldly taking you where many have not dared to tread, accompanied by steaming basmati rice, with scallions for garnish, and sesame seeds for a special textual surprise. A generous serving of asparagus spears and half of an orange, cut into wedges, completes this meal.

1 tablespoon sesame oil

1 teaspoon ginger juice

2 teaspoons Worcestershire sauce, low-sodium

1 teaspoon maple syrup

1 tablespoon red wine

³/₅ block tofu, firm

2½ cups basmati rice, cooked

3 large scallions

1 tablespoon sesame seeds, toasted

Cooking spray

Mix all the marinade ingredients in a large measuring cup: sesame oil, ginger juice, Worcestershire sauce, maple syrup, and red wine. Cut off ⅗ of the tofu block and return the unused portion to the refrigerator for another meal (see below for another idea). Estimate one-third of the remaining tofu and lightly score the top outside corner as a guide. Then cut each of the thirds into two slices. Take the six slices of tofu and place gently into a large ziplock bag. Pour the marinade into the bag, pressing out the excess air, and seal the bag. Marinate overnight in the refrigerator, flipping the bag over whenever you think about it.

Take a nonstick frying pan and coat with a little olive oil. Fry cutlets until nice and crispy on the outside. Serve each person 2 slices of tofu atop a bed of hot rice, covered with 1 scallion sliced thinly, and sprinkled with 1 teaspoon of sesame seeds. This dish would be beautiful paired with asparagus and orange wedges.

YIELD: 3 servings

**Each serving contains approximately:** Calories 312, Fat calories 104, Fat 11.5 g, Saturated fat 1.7 g, Cholesterol 0 mg, Protein 10.3 g, Carbohydrate 30 g, Dietary fiber 1.4 g, Sodium 26 mg, Calories from fat 33%, Calories from saturated fat 5%

**Allowances:** 1⅓ fats + 1 protein + 2¼ starches

# RACHELLE'S STIR-FRY WITH TOFU

This recipe is as individual as you are—make it using the vegetables and seasonings that you like! Remember to prep your vegetables ahead and have cooked brown rice on hand for a quick, delicious, and incredibly healthy and satisfying dinner.

1½ teaspoons canola oil
½ cup red onion, chopped

2 cups bok choy, chopped

1 red bell pepper, chopped

²/₅ block tofu, firm style, cut into cubes

1 cup shiitake mushrooms, sliced

Spices to taste

½ teaspoon sesame oil

1½ cups brown rice, cooked

Heat oil in a wok or a good fry pan. Sauté onions for a few minutes over medium heat. Add the bok choy and bell pepper (or any other vegetables you decide to include) and sauté for another minute or two. Now add the tofu and mushrooms into the mix and start to season! Remove from heat and drizzle toasted sesame oil over the top. Serve over hot rice.

YIELD: 2 servings

**Each serving contains approximately:** Calories 391, Fat calories 90, Fat 10 g, Saturated fat 1 g, Cholesterol 0 mg, Protein 17 g, Carbohydrate 45 g, Dietary fiber 7 g, Sodium 71 mg, Calories from fat 23%, Calories from saturated fat 2%

**Allowances:** 1 fat + 1 protein + 2¼ starches + 3⅔ vegetables

# RACHELLE'S STIR-FRY WITH TOFU AND MONKFISH

This recipe is the same as above, adding in fish.

1½ teaspoons canola oil

½ cup red onion, chopped

1 red bell pepper, chopped

8 ounces monkfish, raw, or 4 ounces shrimp

2 cups bok choy, chopped

²/₅ block tofu, firm style, cut into cubes

1 cup shiitake mushrooms, sliced
Spices to taste
1½ teaspoons sesame oil
1½ cups brown rice, cooked

Heat canola oil in a wok or a good fry pan. Sauté onions for a few minutes over medium heat. Add the peppers and bok choy. Add fish and cook for just a minute. Now, add the tofu and mushrooms into the mix and start to season! Try ground or fresh ginger, a few shakes of the Angostura low-sodium Worcestershire sauce, which has 5 calories and 20 mg sodium per teaspoon (available in the Rice Diet Store and many chain supermarkets), and a pinch of cayenne. You can also use the Mr. Spice Ginger Stir Fry sauce, which has 15 calories and no fat or sodium per tablespoon (at the Rice Diet Store). Remove from heat and drizzle toasted sesame oil over the top. Serve over hot rice.

YIELD: 3 servings

**Each serving contains approximately:** Calories 315, Fat calories 71, Fat 8 g, Saturated fat 1 g, Cholesterol 18 mg, Protein 22 g, Carbohydrate 32 g, Dietary fiber 6 g, Sodium 61 mg, Omega-3 0.3 g, Calories from fat 23%, Calories from saturated fat 3%

**Allowances:** ⅔ fat + 2¼ proteins + 1⅓ starches + 2⅗ vegetables

# RACHELLE'S RICE AND BEANS

This recipe can yield rice and beans for at least four meals, so you have some to put in the freezer. You can easily cut this in half!

2 tablespoons olive oil
2 cups onion, chopped
2 teaspoons cumin

I teaspoon coriander
I teaspoon turmeric
Dash of white pepper
Pinch of red pepper
Black pepper, to taste
I 15-ounce can black beans (Eden)
I 15-ounce can pinto beans (Eden)
2 cans water (30 ounces)
4 cups brown rice, cooked (1½ cup uncooked)

Heat oil in Dutch oven. Sauté onions for a few minutes over medium heat. Add all seasonings and cook 1 or 2 minutes more. Add both cans of beans. Add water to each can and stir to get out remaining beans. Add the two cans of water and bring to a good simmer. Stir in rice. Reseason to suit your taste. Serve with a spoonful of low-fat yogurt, low-fat sour cream, Enrico's Salsa, or Peach Mango Salsa to accent the flavor of this dish. To reheat, just place some beans and rice from the fridge in a microwavable bowl and heat on high for at least 2 minutes to get them good and hot.

YIELD: 12 servings (1 cup per serving)

**Each serving contains approximately:** Calories 161, Fat calories 27, Fat 3 g, Saturated fat 0 g, Cholesterol 0 mg, Protein 6 g, Carbohydrate 29 g, Dietary fiber 5 g, Sodium 13 mg, Calories from fat 17%, Calories from saturated fat 0%

**Allowances:** ½ fat + 1⅔ starches + ⅙ vegetable

# RICE HOUSE LO-MEIN

This Rice House favorite goes well with the *Oriental Salad* (p. 214).

7 ounces spaghetti, cooked
1 teaspoon extra virgin olive oil
1 tablespoon garlic, minced
1 teaspoon ginger
¼ cup snow peas, diced
1 cup bean sprouts
¼ cup green pepper, diced
¼ cup tomato puree, no salt added
¼ cup balsamic vinegar
1 teaspoon sesame seeds
1 pinch wasabi

Cook pasta according to directions on package. Sauté garlic and ginger in olive oil over low-medium heat until garlic is lightly browned. Add ¼ cup water, snow peas, sprouts, and green pepper, and sauté for 2 to 3 minutes. Add tomato puree and vinegar, increase heat to medium, and sauté an additional minute. Fold the pasta into the mixture. If too much liquid is present, reduce heat to low and continue to cook about 1 to 2 minutes or until liquid has evaporated. Add sesame seeds and wasabi just before serving.

YIELD: 6 servings

**Each serving contains approximately:** Calories 158, Fat calories 16, Fat 1.8 g, Saturated fat 0 g, Cholesterol 0 mg, Protein 6 g, Carbohydrate 30 g, Dietary fiber 2 g, Soluble fiber 0 g, Sodium 10 mg, Calories from fat 10%, Calories from saturated fat 0%

**Allowances:** ⅙ fat + 1⅗ starches + ½ vegetable

# BAKED SALMON WITH HONEY MUSTARD BED

At the Rice House, Chef J.R. prefers to serve this salmon dish over rice to maximize the flavor from the juice created by the honey-mustard sauce.

6 6-ounce salmon fillets
I cup lemon juice, freshly squeezed
½ cup dry mustard
4 tablespoons honey
I teaspoon black pepper
2 tablespoons garlic, minced
2 tablespoons parsley, freshly chopped

Preheat oven to 350 degrees F. Place salmon in 2-inch-deep baking pan, add 1 cup of water and 1 cup lemon juice. Cover and bake for 15 to 20 minutes. Take a large saucepan and place 1½ cups of water on high heat. After water boils, add mustard and stir fast. Slowly add honey, black pepper, and garlic. Set on low heat and stir every 2 to 3 minutes until fish is done. Take fish out of pan and pour juice from pan into saucepan. Stir on medium heat for 5 minutes. Spoon 1 ounce of mustard sauce on plate, place salmon on top, add parsley, and serve!

YIELD: 6 servings

**Each serving contains approximately:** Calories 374, Fat calories 153, Fat 17 g, Saturated fat 2 g, Cholesterol 99 mg, Protein 35 g, Carbohydrate 20 g, Dietary fiber 1 g, Sodium 81 mg, Omega-3 2 g, Calories from fat 41%, Calories from saturated fat 5%

**Allowances:** ⅔ starch + 5 proteins

# CRISPY FLOUNDER

The delicate flavor of the fish is enhanced by the subtle breading and spices to create a scrumptious main course.

6 6-ounce flounder fillets
¼ cup lemon juice
1 teaspoon extra virgin olive oil
1 Toufayan Salt Free Pita, diced
½ cup Roma tomatoes, diced
½ cup onion, diced
1 teaspoon garlic, minced
1 teaspoon black pepper
1 teaspoon fresh basil
½ teaspoon oregano, freshly chopped
½ teaspoon cayenne pepper
1 tablespoon parsley, freshly chopped

Marinate fish in lemon juice mixed with ¼ cup water. Preheat oven to 350 degrees F. Set fillets in a shallow olive oil–coated baking pan. Combine remaining ingredients (except parsley) to form a type of batter. Lightly pat the mixture over the fish. Pour the water/lemon juice marinade around—not on—the fillets. Cover and bake for 15 to 17 minutes. Uncover, switch oven to broil, and cook another 1 to 2 minutes or until top begins to brown. Top with fresh parsley and serve.

YIELD: 6 servings

**Each serving contains approximately:** Calories 179, Fat calories 26, Fat 2.9 g, Saturated fat 0.6 g, Cholesterol 82 mg, Protein 33 g, Carbohydrate 6 g, Dietary fiber 0.5 g, Sodium 140 mg, Omega-3 0.4 g, Calories from fat 15%, Calories from saturated fat 3%

**Allowances:** ⅙ fat + 3 proteins + ⅙ vegetable

# FISH STEW

So simple yet so delicious—and so low fat! Pair this with a bruschetta and you will be transported!

1 tablespoon extra virgin olive oil
1 large onion, thinly sliced
2 garlic cloves, thinly sliced
1 cup dry white wine
1 28-ounce can crushed tomatoes, no salt added
Freshly ground pepper, as desired
1 pound tuna fillet
1 pound swordfish fillet
1 pound medium shrimp, peeled and deveined
¼ cup Italian parsley, roughly chopped
1 teaspoon oregano, chopped

In a large, heavy-bottomed saucepan, warm the olive oil over medium heat. Add the onion and garlic and sauté until the onion is translucent. Add the wine and tomato, season with pepper, and cook for 30 minutes, stirring occasionally. Add the tuna, swordfish, and shrimp, and cook for 10 to 15 minutes, or until all the seafood is cooked through, stirring occasionally. Adjust the seasoning; stir in the parsley and oregano and serve.

YIELD: 6 servings

**Each serving contains approximately:** Calories 323, Fat Calories 61, Fat 7 g, Saturated fat 1 g, Cholesterol 173 mg, Protein 45 g, Carbohydrates 11 g, Dietary fiber 3 g, Sodium 240 mg, Omega-3 2 g, Calories from fat 19%, Calories from saturated fat 3%

**Allowances:** ½ fat + 6½ proteins + 1⅜ vegetables

# LOBSTER BISQUE

This is one of Kitty's favorite dishes that we reserve for special occasions. It's rich and flavorful. And, by all means, you can use frozen lobster tails!

6 lobster tails
6 cups fish stock (3 8-ounce tubs of Perfect Additions no-salt-added
    Rich Fish Stock plus 24 ounces water, as directed)
1 onion
1 carrot
1 fennel bulb (celery can be substituted)
1 tablespoon extra virgin olive oil
2 tablespoons tomato paste, no salt added
½ cup brandy
2 cups evaporated skim milk

Remove the lobster meat from the shell. This is best done by using scissors to cut the belly membrane where it joins the shell from each side or by splitting the shell with a heavy knife. The meat should be diced and set aside. The shell should be cut into 1- to 2-inch pieces.

Reconstitute the fish broth with the water in a saucepan on medium heat. Cut onion, carrot, and fennel bulb into 1-inch pieces. Heat 2 teaspoons of olive oil in a heavy pot over high heat. Add onion, carrot, and fennel pieces in the pot, and cook until they begin to color. Use a little fish stock, if needed, to keep sauté from sticking.

Turn down the heat to medium. Add the lobster shells and cook until they begin to color. Add the tomato paste and mix thoroughly, letting it caramelize. Carefully add the brandy and light with a taper. When the flash of flame dies, add in fish broth and simmer for 45 minutes. Strain the vegetables and shells out of the broth and continue to simmer the broth.

Heat the remaining teaspoon of olive oil in a nonstick pan. Add the lobster meat and cook until just opaque. Transfer the almost-cooked lobster meat into the broth. Add the evaporated skim milk and stir for 2 minutes.

YIELD: 6 servings

**Each serving contains approximately:** Calories 281, Fat calories 56, Fat 6 g, Saturated fat 1 g, Cholesterol 143 mg, Protein 34 g, Carbohydrate 13 g, Dietary fiber 2 g, Sodium 552 mg, Omega-3 0.8 g, Calories from fat 20%, Calories from saturated fat 3%

**Allowances:** ½ fat + 3½ proteins + ⅔ dairy + ¼ vegetable

# MARINATED SWORDFISH

This is another delicious way to enjoy swordfish. You can use the marinade to cook the fish in or use it as a topping when serving the dish at room temperature for a Sunday lunch.

6 garlic cloves, fresh, thinly sliced
½ cup oregano leaves (loosely packed), or 2 tablespoons freshly
    chopped Italian parsley
¼ cup red wine vinegar
½ cup extra virgin olive oil
¼ cup lemon juice, freshly squeezed
Black pepper, freshly ground, to taste
4 swordfish steaks, ½-inch thick (about 2 pounds)

In a small bowl combine the garlic, oregano, vinegar, ¼ cup of water, oil, and lemon juice, and season with several grinds of black pepper. Pour half of the marinade into a small pitcher. Use half to brush the fish before cooking and the other half after cooking.

Prepare grill. Brush fish lightly with the marinade and put on the grill. Cook until fish is lightly golden, approximately 2 minutes each side. Place fish in a large shallow dish that can accommodate the fish in one layer. Marinate for about 1 hour at room temperature, basting a few times.

Yield: 4 servings

**Each serving contains approximately:** Calories 360, Fat calories 147, Total fat 17 g, Saturated fat 2.4 g, Cholesterol 86 mg, Protein 42 g, Carbohydrates 2 g, Dietary fiber 0 g, Sodium 205 mg, Omega-3 2 g, Calories from fat 42%, Calories from saturated fat 10%

**Allowances:** 2 fats + 6 proteins + ⅛ vegetable

NOTE: Calculations made by estimating one-quarter of marinade consumed.

# SEAFOOD GUMBO

Rice House Chef J.R. recommends serving this spicy gumbo over rice—just like in Cajun country.

¼ cup lemon juice
6 ounces grouper, cleaned and quartered
6 ounces flounder, cleaned and quartered
6 ounces salmon, cleaned and quartered
1 teaspoon olive oil
2 teaspoons garlic, minced
1 cup onion, diced
1 whole potato, skinned and cubed
½ cup corn
½ cup peas
¼ cup tomato puree, no salt added
¼ cup yellow squash, cubed
¼ cup zucchini, cubed
1 tablespoon honey
1 pinch black pepper
1 pinch oregano
1 pinch fresh basil
1 pinch gumbo filé

Marinate fish in lemon juice. In a pot, sauté garlic and onion in olive oil until lightly browned. Add 3 cups of water, increase heat to medium, add vegetables and spices, cover, and simmer 3 to 4 minutes. Stir in fish, add more water if necessary, increase heat, and bring to a light boil. Boil 2 to 3 minutes, reduce heat to medium-low, cover, and cook 5 to 6 minutes or until fish flakes easily with a fork.

YIELD: 6 servings

**Each serving contains approximately:** Calories 192, Fat calories 44, Fat 4.9 g, Saturated fat 0.9 g, Cholesterol 41 mg, Protein 18 g, Carbohydrates 19 g, Dietary fiber 2 g, Sodium 62 mg, Omega-3 0.7 g, Calories from fat 23%, Calories from saturated fat 4%

**Allowances:** ⅙ fat + 2⅓ proteins + ⅔ starch + ½ vegetable

# LEMON SHRIMP

This shrimp dish is bursting with lemon flavor.

1 tablespoon extra virgin olive oil
¾ pound medium shrimp, peeled and deveined
Pinch red chili pepper flakes
3 garlic cloves, sliced
¼ cup limoncello or other citrus liqueur
1 lemon, zest and juice
½ cup parsley leaves, chopped
4 slices no-salt-added bread

Heat oil, shrimp, chili pepper flakes, and garlic in frying pan over medium high heat. When garlic starts to brown add limoncello. When most of the liquid has evaporated, remove from heat and add lemon juice, zest, and parsley. Toast the bread, then spread the shrimp on toast and serve.

NOTE: This can also be tossed with pasta.

YIELD: 4 servings

**Each serving contains approximately:** Calories 138, Fat calories 36, Fat 4 g, Saturated fat 0.5 g, Cholesterol 32 mg, Protein 7 g, Carbohydrate 20 g, Dietary fiber 1 g, Omega-3 0.6 g, Sodium 39 mg, Calories from fat 26%, Calories from saturated fat 3%

**Allowances:** ¾ fat + 1 protein + 1 starch + ¼ fruit

# DIAMANT INSPIRED HALIBUT

A participant inspired this recipe during one of Rachelle's cooking classes.

2 teaspoons olive oil
2 tablespoons shallots, thinly sliced
½ red bell pepper, medium, sliced
1 8-ounce halibut fillet, without skin, cut into large cubes
Freshly ground black pepper, plenty
Pinch of cayenne pepper
1 teaspoon turmeric
½ teaspoon cumin
½ cup vegetable bouillon (make extra)
2 teaspoons Angostura Worcestershire sauce, low-sodium
Juice from ½ lemon

Heat oil in a saucepan over medium heat. Add shallots and red pepper and sauté for a minute or two. Add halibut and spices and sauté for another minute or two. The fish will break apart some but this is all right. Add bouillon and Worcestershire sauce and lift up any of the fish that has begun to stick to the pan. Add more bouillon if necessary with the reserve. Taste the broth and reseason to suite your preference. Serve in a bowl over rice if you like. Squeeze fresh lemon juice over the top.

YIELD: 2 servings

**Each serving contains approximately:** Calories 235, Fat calories 70, Fat 7.7 g, Saturated fat 1 g, Cholesterol 47 mg, Protein 32 g, Carbohydrate 6 g, Dietary fiber 1 g, Omega-3s 0.59 g, Sodium 133 mg, Calories from fat 30%, Calories from saturated fat 4%

**Allowances:** 1 fat + 3 proteins + 1 vegetable

# RACHELLE'S ENCRUSTED BAKED TUNA

This is a delicious way to enjoy tuna. You can add any low-sodium seasoning you want here (e.g., tarragon, thyme, rosemary, black pepper, or red pepper). Place the baked fish on top of a bed of salad greens along with some type of fruit and you have a complete and lovely meal.

1 10-ounce tuna fillet, skinless, cut in two pieces
¼ cup soy milk
2 Ryvita Sesame Rye crisp breads (crumbled)
12 almonds, roasted and chopped
1 teaspoon sesame seeds
Herbs and spices, to taste

Make sure fish is dry. Add soy milk to a plate or flat dish. Dip each piece of fish into soy milk and drag through on both sides. Coat fish completely in the crisp bread crumbs, almonds, and sesame seeds. Place on a nonstick baking sheet or use parchment paper. Season top with herbs and spices. Place in preheated 375 to 400 degrees F oven for about 10 to 12 minutes. You might want to flip the oven over to low broil just at the end to brown the top nicely. Be sure to watch the fish carefully, especially if browning the top.

YIELD: 2 servings

**Each serving contains approximately:** Calories 281, Fat calories 90, Fat 10 g, Saturated fat 1 g, Cholesterol 63 mg, Protein 37 g, Carbohydrate 12 g, Dietary fiber 3 g, Omega-3 0.34 g, Sodium 114 mg, Calories from fat 32%, Calories from saturated fat 3%

**Allowances:** ½ fat + 4 proteins + ½ starch

# RACHELLE'S ENCRUSTED HALIBUT WITH QUINOA PILAF

The halibut and quinoa blend together for a rich taste and texture.

ENCRUSTED HALIBUT

1 8-ounce halibut fillet, skinless
1 egg white
2 Ryvita Sesame Rye crisp breads (crumbled)
Herbs and spices, to taste

QUINOA APRICOT PILAF

1½ cups Red Inca quinoa, cooked
½ cup apricot juice
5 apricots, dried, sliced

Make sure fish is dry. Cut fillet evenly in half widthwise. Dip in egg white. Coat fish completely in the crisp bread crumbs. Place on a nonstick baking sheet or use parchment paper. Season top with herbs and spices. Place in preheated 375 degrees F oven for about 10 to 12 minutes. You might want to flip the oven over to low broil just at the end to brown the top nicely. Be sure to watch the fish carefully, especially if browning the top.

Make the quinoa per directions (be sure to rinse under hot water to remove the bitter taste before cooking). Heat up nonstick skillet and add apricot juice. Add apricot slices and allow to warm and expand for a minute. Add quinoa when apricot juice is hot and mix together. The liquid will either be absorbed by the quinoa or evaporate off. Take off heat before quinoa dries out and serve. Think about making this apricot quinoa pilaf alone as a dish to accompany any other entrée.

Use a sprig of rosemary or thyme as garnish for the fish. Experiment and enjoy!

YIELD: 2 servings

**Each serving contains approximately:** Calories 350, Fat calories 72, Fat 8 g, Saturated fat 0.6 g, Cholesterol 47 mg, Protein 43 g, Carbohydrate 27 g, Dietary fiber 9 g, Omega-3 0.59 g, Sodium 135 mg, Calories from fat 13%, Calories from saturated fat 1%

**Allowances:** 3 proteins + 2 starches + 1¼ fruits

# SCAMPI

This shrimp dish is quick and simple but packed with lemony flavor. It's also excellent over rice, risotto, or polenta.

7 ounces pasta
1 teaspoon extra virgin olive oil
8 ounces shrimp, large (31–35), cleaned and shelled
4 garlic cloves, sliced thinly
1 teaspoon black pepper
¼ cup white wine
¼ cup lemon juice, fresh
1 tablespoon fresh parsley, chopped

Cook pasta according to directions on package. Heat olive oil in large fry pan and add shrimp, garlic, and pepper. Sauté until shrimp curls. Remove from heat, add wine, and place back on heat. Simmer for 1 to 2 minutes. Cover pan and place on high heat. Wait 1 minute.

Remove cover, stir well, plate, and top with lemon juice and fresh parsley.

Yᴉᴇʟᴅ: 4 servings

**Each serving contains approximately:** Calories 230, Fat calories 18, Fat 2 g, Saturated fat 0 g, Cholesterol 42 mg, Protein 12 g, Carbohydrate 40 g, Dietary fiber 4 g, Omega-3 0.3 g, Sodium 28 mg, Calories from fat 7%, Calories from saturated fat 0%

**Allowances:** ¼ fat + 2¼ starches + 1¼ protein

# TREATS

Desserts can be delicious and low in fat. Here are some Rice House favorites.

## BLUEBERRY-PEACH COBBLER

This cobbler just melts in your mouth.

1 teaspoon extra virgin olive oil
1 cup fresh blueberries
2 cups fresh peaches, peeled and cut into bite-size pieces
6 teaspoons flaxseed, ground
1 cup oatmeal, raw
1 tablespoon vanilla extract
2 teaspoons cinnamon

Preheat oven to 450 degrees F. Coat a small 2-inch-deep baking pan with olive oil. Place blueberries and peaches in pan. In a coffee grinder or blender, finely grind the flaxseed and then mix with remaining ingredients. Add mixture to fruit and stir well to combine. Bake about 25 minutes. Serve cool or warm.

YIELD: 6 servings

**Each serving contains approximately:** Calories 116, Fat calories 27, Fat 3 g, Saturated fat 0.5 g, Cholesterol 0 mg, Protein 3 g, Carbohydrate 20 g, Dietary fiber 4 g, Sodium 4 mg, Calories from fat 23%, Calories from saturated fat 4%

**Allowances:** ⅙ fat + ¾ starch + ¾ fruit

# BLUEBERRY-BANANA MUFFINS

Chef Nancy whips up this muffin batter with all sorts of fruit. You can substitute the blueberries with whatever is in season. You can also bake the batter on a sheet and enjoy it as a bread.

3 bananas
½ cup pears, canned
1 tablespoon cinnamon
1 tablespoon vanilla extract
½ cup fresh blueberries
1½ cups oatmeal, uncooked
1 teaspoon olive oil

Preheat oven to 450 degrees F. Mash bananas and pears in a large bowl. Add cinnamon and vanilla and mix well. Fold in blueberries and oatmeal. Thinly coat muffin pan with olive oil. Pour batter into muffin pan and bake for 30 to 45 minutes.

YIELD: 6 servings (1 muffin per serving)

**Each serving contains approximately:** Calories 155, Fat calories 18, Fat 2 g, Saturated fat 0 g, Cholesterol 0 mg, Protein 4 g, Carbohydrate 33 g, Dietary fiber 5 g, Sodium 3 mg, Calories from fat 12%, Calories from saturated fat 0%

**Allowances:** 1 starch + 1¼ fruits

# CLEMENTINES AND STRAWBERRIES WITH VINEGAR AND PEPPER

Clementines are small but packed with flavor. Enjoy this dish as a salad with your meal or as a spicy dessert.

8 clementines (you can substitute other small seedless citrus)
2 cups fresh strawberries
2 ounces balsamic vinegar (the best you can find)
1 teaspoon honey
Freshly ground black pepper

Peel the clementines and separate them into segments. Combine with the strawberries, vinegar, honey, and fresh pepper.

YIELD: 4 servings

**Each serving contains approximately:** Calories 122, Fat calories 3, Fat 0.5 g, Saturated fat 0 g, Cholesterol 0 mg, Protein 2 g, Carbohydrate 30 g, Dietary fiber 6 g, Sodium 2 mg, Calories from fat 3%, Calories from saturated fat 0%

**Allowances:** 1/10 starch + 3/4 fruits

# GRILLED PEACHES

Have you ever thought of grilling fruit? Try it, you'll LOVE it!

4 local peaches
1 teaspoon extra virgin olive oil
1/4 teaspoon freshly ground black pepper

Cut peaches in half and remove pits. Coat peaches with a little oil, place on broiling pan skin side down, and lightly grind a turn or two of black pepper on each inner surface.

YIELD: 4 servings

**Each serving contains approximately:** Calories 53, Fat calories 11, Fat 1 g, Saturated fat 0 g, Cholesterol 0 mg, Protein 1 g, Carbohydrate 11 g, Dietary fiber 2 g, Sodium 0 mg, Calories from fat 20%, Calories from saturated fat 0%

**Allowances:** ¼ fat + ¾ fruit

# SWEET POTATO PIE

Chef Nancy serves this Rice House favorite in the fall when sweet potatoes are in season.

4 sweet potatoes
1 banana
½ cup prunes, chopped
½ cup pineapple, chopped
1 teaspoon cinnamon
2 tablespoons flaxseed, ground in a coffee mill or blender
1 teaspoon vanilla extract

Preheat oven to 450 degrees F. Bake sweet potatoes for 45 to 55 minutes, allow to cool, then peel. Mash sweet potatoes and banana in a mixing bowl. Whisk in prunes, pineapple, cinnamon, flaxseed, and vanilla extract. Mixture will have a creamy texture. Spread mixture in an 8 x 8–inch pan and bake for 25 minutes.

YIELD: 6 servings

**Each serving contains approximately:** Calories 174, Fat calories 41, Fat 4.6 g, Saturated fat 0.5 g, Cholesterol 0 mg, Protein 2 g, Carbohydrate 34 g, Dietary fiber 4 g, Sodium 31 mg, Calories from fat 24%, Calories from saturated fat 3%

**Allowances:** ⅛ fat + 1 starch + ⅞ fruit

# ORANGE DREAM

This recipe was inspired by the *New Mayo Clinic Cookbook* (Ox-moor House, 2004). Whip up this frothy cooler in seconds—it tastes like an old-fashioned creamsicle. For best results, start with ice-cold soy milk, and use freshly squeezed orange juice. Creamy, custardlike silken tofu adds extra body.

1½ cups orange juice, freshly squeezed
1 cup vanilla soy milk, chilled
⅓ cup tofu, silken or soft
1 teaspoon orange zest
½ teaspoon vanilla extract
5 ice cubes
1 orange, peeled
4 mint sprigs

In a blender, combine the orange juice, soy milk, tofu, half the orange and its zest, vanilla, and ice cubes. Blend until smooth and frothy, about 30 seconds. Pour into tall, chilled glasses and garnish each glass with an orange segment and a sprig of mint.

YIELD: 4 servings

**Each serving contains approximately:** Calories 105, Fat calories 9, Fat 1 g, Saturated fat 0 g, Cholesterol 0 mg, Protein 4 g, Carbohydrate 20 g, Dietary fiber 0 g, Sodium 56 mg, Calories from fat 9%, Calories from saturated fat 0%

**Allowances:** ½ dairy + ¼ starch + ¾ fruit

# QUINOA PUDDING

Enjoy this versatile pudding for breakfast, brunch, snack, or dessert.

1 cup quinoa
2 cups boiling water
⅓ cup raisins or dried cherries
½ cup unsweetened apple juice
2 bananas
⅓ teaspoon lemon rind, grated
¾ teaspoon lemon juice, freshly squeezed
1 teaspoon vanilla
½ teaspoon cinnamon

Rinse quinoa in hot water and drain while waiting for water to boil. This is an important step since quinoa contains a phytochemical called saponin, which has a bitter taste if not well rinsed. Add quinoa to boiling water, then reduce heat to medium-low. Boil quinoa for 10 minutes, then add raisins or dried cherries and boil for another 5 minutes. While quinoa is cooking, put remaining ingredients in a blender or food processor and blend until smooth. Add the blended ingredients into the quinoa and simmer for 5 more minutes, or until desired consistency is achieved.

YIELD: 4 servings (¾ cup per serving)

**Each serving contains approximately:** Calories 230, Fat calories 27, Fat 2.9 g, Saturated fat 0.7 g, Cholesterol 0 mg, Protein 6 g, Carbohydrate 51 g, Dietary fiber 5 g, Sodium 20 mg, Calories from fat 11%, Calories from saturated fat 0%

**Allowances:** 1⅓ starches + 1⅚ fruits

# FINAL NOTE

D reams, or desires of our heart, do come to fruition when we persevere and continue to move toward our goal. This book is an example of a dream that has been "on my heart," then "in my womb" for years. It was more similar to birthing our 10-pound, 1-ounce baby than anything I can compare it to. I felt its inevitableness; it being part of my "package" (as Agnes Sanford would call it), which includes being "giftlike" and divine in essence, as well as uniquely my responsibility, like a calling or a mission to fulfill. Various paths and passageways led to this final product, or handbook for healing, that may inspire you on your own. Because even though we are all partaking in different learning opportunities, and thus need and create different journeys, we certainly can glean from another's pain, miseries, miracles, and healings.

The Rice Diet is about healing. It's first about healing the body, most often of its overweight and resulting health conditions. And then it's about healing the mind and spirit. We are all creating unhealthy and largely unconscious responses in our bodies. When some people get stressed or lonely they have a "hand-to-mouth-with-food" response to soothe themselves, while others send more loaded neurological and hormonal-inspired stress responses to their joints (arthritis), muscles (back pain), guts (ulcers, irritable bowel syndrome), and to their brains (headaches, migraines). The good news is that we all have the potential and power to be healthier and happier by making conscious choices, and this process means taking the steps to discover the path to our own inner healing.

Of course, there are as many paths to healing as there are individuals in the world. Some people pursue a spiritual answer to their problems. They seek to know themselves by connecting to the Creative Source of the universe that resides within us all, through activities such as yoga, tai chi, mindfulness meditation, prayers, and journalizing.

Others find the key to their inner healing through support in the community of others, since much of our emotional pain and resulting physical disease is due to our struggle to communicate and realize our need to love and connect with others. Bob and I have witnessed this again and again with participants at the Rice Diet program. The participants who have seemed to experience the most dramatic healing of a shame-based past were the ones who described how much they have come to love and accept themselves. Although this may sound overly simplistic, Thich Naht Hanh's reminder to "water the good seeds" comes to mind. Rather than continue to keep company with the same degrading forces that put you down or push high fat, salt, and sugar foods toward you, make some new empowering, affirming friends that habitually water the good seeds of healing, transformation, and actualization of your dreams. There are plenty of others out there seeking community with other positive people seeking to maximize their potential. I believe that if you open yourself to the opportunity to meet encouraging people, who do not have a lifelong habit of judging and blaming you for not being as thin as they desire you to be, they will come.

And there are still other people who make the healing connection by learning about the science behind why we don't do what we really want to do with our lives and health. There has been a recent explosion of fascinating research in this arena. The newly discovered role of the old brain, the amygdala, can be pivotal in understanding ourselves and our behavior when our impulsive feelings override our rational mind. Incoming messages come from the senses, and the amygdala scans them for potential trouble. This primitive, fastest responding part of the brain is geared to react quickly to save us from the likes of the copperhead snake that bit and harmed our neighbor last year. So if our brain receives the message that a snakelike object is near our foot, the amygdala will have us running long before our rational brain investigates the exact type of snake, and thus the degree of danger we are confronting. Likewise, if someone hurts our feelings, many of us will "run away" from the pain by downing a good brownie or ice-cream cone. We reach for the brownie so quickly that we don't even give ourselves a second to remember the recent commitment to our *dieta* that has given us back our life. When people understand how they might be responding addictively to stress by turning to food, they are able to begin to make different choices that eventually will retrain the neuronal pathways and the amygdala.

In the film, *What the Bleep Do We Know?* (Lord of the Wind Films, 2004), and its companion book *The Little Book of Bleeps*, some of the world's most esteemed physicists discuss how quantum physics research has proven that neuronal synapses that are not acted upon, but that instead start firing in another direction, will develop a greater tendency to repeat on the most frequented path. In other words, we can become conscious of our knee-jerk reactions with food, and consciously choose to replace them, repeatedly, with more health-promoting responses. The more we do this, the greater the likelihood that these new responses will become our so-called habit energy and thus enhance our odds to respond to stress by taking a nice brisk walk or bath, or secluding ourselves with a journal or meditation tape or Bible, and releasing our frustrations in healthier ways.

The Rice Diet encompasses all these tools—intellectual education, inner self-reflection, community support, and of course, the diet itself, which leads you to eat clean, whole foods that inspire detoxification, weight loss, and health. All these tools work synergistically: the health-promoting *dieta* includes not only the cleansing optimal diet, but the renewed energy and clarity to retain the education on nutrition and psycho-neuro-immunology (how the mind, body, and immunity, thus health, are connected), which then fuels the openness for the inner healing and your emotional and spiritual personal journey.

But I have found that there is one simple key that opens the door

to all these paths to healing: you have to be open and willing to receive the truth, whatever it is. I know this firsthand. Up until New
Year's Day, 1989, I believed that if you were a nonsmoking, semiveg-
etarian athlete, you were bulletproof from chronic disease. Then one
morning I awoke to find myself crippled with a joint disorder so profound that I could barely walk.

I went to see doctors; I did my own research, but it was not until
I saw and accepted the truth about my illness that I was able to heal
and be healed. To make a long, complicated story short, I became
aware that the root cause of my illness was resentment that I had
been harboring and carrying around within me. The power of this
realization was revealed when a friend who I hadn't seen in years
stayed over at our house the night before I awoke crippled. When I
entered the kitchen from my room, he entered at the same moment
from the living room. As soon as he saw my look of fear and heard
my description of crippling pain, he said that he knew that I would
be healed as soon as I allowed God to heal my resentment. Sam is an
Episcopal priest who is gifted with healing and wisdom. It was one
of the only times in my life that I have been speechless; there were
no words to follow that direct a truth.

The good news was that in that moment I was given the faith and
blessed assurance that I was going to be healed. The overwhelming
news was that in that moment I also knew my healing was dependent upon my choice to perceive things differently, to let go of the
false belief that I was supposed to be in control of far more than I
was and let go of my pent-up resentment. Specifically, I was waking
up every morning with my fists clenched because I was taking it personally that the administration where I worked did not prioritize my
heart disease reversal plan for our cardiac patients. And it is probably easy for you, at your vantage point, to see how this stressful
physiological response was obviously not facilitating my desired
agenda. But, when a triathlete, who's been a vegetarian for fifteen
years, hits the wall—not due to carbohydrate depletion, but due to
an intense and dramatic realization that my emotional, mental, and
spiritual state, and responses were largely responsible for my crip-

pling joint condition, it was devastating. It was my first awareness that I actually could create such pain and disease in my life, and that I also can control the pain and co-create the life I desire. It was at that moment that I chose to become more conscious of any unhealthy response I was having, to perceive and respond differently, to respond out of love rather than fear, and to open myself to a healing of the emotional and spiritual underpinnings of the physical disease I was manifesting. I knew I would be totally healed, but the journey seemed long and periodically terrifying.

When I look back to that time the word that comes to mind is "precession." Buckminister (Bucky) Fuller, one of my favorite renaissance men of this last century, coined the word "precession" as moving toward what feels right to you and staying focused on what delights you. It is best illustrated by the honeybee who passionately pursues the flower, the essence of what he desires, having no idea that in doing so he is fulfilling the true purpose in his life. He also has no idea that without him being who he is here to be, life as we know it would be forever radically changed, if not extinguished! He just does what he feels led to do, and by simply doing this, without getting overly analytical, critical, fearful, or constipated about his success, he fulfills his true purpose in life. Bucky would finish his discussion on precession by saying that if a person remains steadfast to his true purpose and goals, then the Great Spirit will provide at the last possible moment. Well, that's what happened; I continued to do what felt right to do next, and God's spirit finally moved, and I was totally healed.

As I share my belief that resentment was the root cause of my crippling joint disorder, I do so to inspire others to examine and explore possible emotional and spiritual underpinnings of their own physical diseases, including their weight problem. Some people have expressed how inviting others to look at what responsibility they may have in "co-creating" their disease may bring up shame and blame responses, rather than empowering breakthroughs and healing. This is of some concern as many overeating addicted persons have expressed how they feel that being shamed as a child by their parents was a root cause of their weight and body image problems. For readers that share this pain from shame, I invite you to seek a highly recommended overeating therapist near you, a loving and confidential support group to encourage your weight loss and healing goals (OA, ACOA, or other groups supportive of your physical, emotional, and spiritual goals), and a beautiful journal to encourage your daily journalizing of feelings that come up as you make this new commitment to yourself and your life.

The dramatic and miraculous healing of this arthritic-like condition taught me many, many things, especially the belief that all of our answers and potential for healing are already within us. When people take the time to slow down, be honest with themselves and others, open themselves to the growing pains suffered and wisdom gleaned from others, and learn to listen to others with an open heart and mind—without an agenda to fix or change them, while getting really conscious and aware of what is coming out of their mouths and the mouths of their fellow community members—many are healed. When participants hear a thin, athletic, vegetarian dietitian honestly share how she struggled with a control addiction, resulting resentment habit, and arthritic-like pain for nine months, and was healed via her invitation to the creative force of the universe to move through her commitment to the inner healing process, participants shift. I can see and feel how they move from their prior judgment of me as "having it easier than them," because I "inherited a high metabolism or gene for thinness" to realizing, "Wow, she's as flawed as me," or "She's just carried her pain in different ways."

One Ricer comes to mind, a man I will call David. At a meeting, David began introducing himself to the group, as he had for each weekly group in the year he had been there. He said what he had always said, which was, "My name is David and my doctor said I should be dead."

He would add a few sentences justifying how serious his heart condition was and how the doctors said there was no hope for him; and he would finish with an endearing and appreciative mini-commercial of gratitude for our staff that had saved his life. I had previously listened to him share this same summary each week, thinking that I would not push him to go deeper than he felt comfortable. But one day, I asked him from my heart, "David, how is it serving you to repeat that others believe you should be dead?" He squirmed and meekly defended his story that these brilliant doctors, who knew far more than he did, had no idea how he was still alive.

I then asked him what *he* believed . . . and what *his experience was* . . . and kept asking him leading questions to explore why *he remained so identified with his survival position.* He stayed with me in this loving and honest exchange for about twenty minutes. I will always remember it as one of the holiest, most honest and significant communications I have ever had with another being. I could tell he did not sense any attack from me, but was honored that I loved him enough to be so truly honest with him—despite the risk of others present.

After the group, he came up to me, closer than he ever had before, within inches of my face, and said, "Kitty, I think I've got it! My repeating that I should be dead is probably more damaging to my health than eating sodium is to my congestive heart failure!" I put my hands on either side of his face, and said, "You got it all right! David, I will resist the temptation to kiss you on the mouth!"

When he first came, he couldn't walk the ten steps from the handicapped parking place to the blood pressure station; one and a half years later he was walking six to eight miles per day, challenging others to keep up, and spreading gratitude everywhere he trekked. His love and gratitude for life and others was the ultimate reminder that it is not the length of our life but the love given and received that is most important.

A few life-packed months later David died on the trail, his favorite woodsy walk, on a glorious, sunny Carolina spring day, exiting just as he would have had it. Our community was stunned and shocked. Despite our knowing how sick he was, he no longer appeared to be. He epitomized the super-energized life of a resurrected man. Despite how very sick David was, he will always be remembered as the most grateful man there. And as he resurrected and began to feel better and better himself, he spread it around to others, always eager to cheerlead or command others to their highest.

David would have wanted me to seriously challenge you to take your life on—to really commit to the *Rice Dieta*. David really "got" the transformation potential of fasting from anything man-made. We were designed to eat food, not pharmaceuticals! I know this is anecdotal and there is no scientific proof that people get more insightful, introspective, and aware of what they are doing, feeling, and thinking on a no-salt-added, vegetarian diet, but I challenge you to try it for yourself. Of course, in addition to the ultra-clean dietary aspects, the *Rice Dieta* encompasses the lifestyle choices that assist you in slowing down, assessing your dreams and feelings about where you are and where you want to go with the co-creation of your life. How the *dieta* affects you personally is more important and convincing than anything we could say or research; so do yourself and the world a favor, and commit to it.

If you knew you had five years to live the life of your dreams, what would that look like? I challenge you to take your journal and spend the next hour answering that question. Take off the top, your lid or blinders, and answer it with no limitations, answering it "as if" you are guaranteed of not failing. No kidding. Considering how much what we believe shapes our life's opinions and potential, really allow yourself to write your wildest dreams and really express what you want to do with the rest of your life. When you truly get in touch with what matters to you it is often surprising. Your dreams may start off with big goals like "make a difference in creating world peace," and then get more personal and specific, like "heal the broken relationship with my son and create a great connection with his son." This may lead to more simple or important details like, "I will reach my goal weight and regain the balance and health to bicycle on the beach road with my grandson each week. It will be the greatest gift I can give my son . . . and his." It's this kind of honesty and clarity that inspires people to get clear on what is important to them, to tap into a level of consciousness that transforms them into lasting commitments that create new neuronal circuitry. Here's to standing as a source for a transformed world . . . that begins with you.

# APPENDIX A

## Mail-Order Sources for Health Foods

Some of the delicious and healthy products mentioned in this book may be difficult for you to obtain in your community. The following information will assist you in contacting the companies directly to request information on their products, ordering procedures, and costs.

## BASICS

Rice Diet Store
1644 Cole Mill Road
Durham, NC 27705
(919) 383-7276, ext. 2
www.ricedietstore.com

The Rice Diet Store carries pantry staples such as grains, beans, and cereals, as well as gourmet items, including a selection of the finest imported olive oils and vinegars. All foods have been carefully selected by our nutrition staff and adhere to our standards for great-tasting, low-sodium foods.

# BREAD OR BAKED GOODS

Toufayan Bakeries, Inc.
175 Railroad Avenue
Ridgefield, NJ 07657
(800) 328-7482
www.toufayan.com

or

Toufayan Bakeries, Inc.
3826 Bryn Mawr Street
Orlando, FL 32808
(800) 233-7482

Toufayan makes 8-ounce salt-free white and whole wheat pitas. Their pita bread products, called Pitettes, measure 3½ by 4 inches in diameter and freeze beautifully. The Web site includes a complete product list, recipes, and contact information. If Toufayan products are not available in your area, they will gladly ship via UPS.

Food For Life Baking Company (Ezekiel 4:9 Bread)
PO Box 1434
Corona, CA 92878
www.foodforlife.com

Food For Life Baking Company, makers of the fabulous Ezekiel 4:9 Breads, is a family-owned and -operated specialty bakery with a passionate commitment to natural foods. Among the products specifically developed to meet particular dietary requirements are two organic sprouted-grain, low-sodium breads. Access their Web site to find a retail store near you.

# FRESH FRUIT

If you can't buy organic produce locally, the following companies supply organic fresh fruit year-round.

Cushman Fruit Company
3325 Forest Hill Blvd.
West Palm Beach, FL 33406
(800) 776-7575
www.honeybell.com

Mack's Groves
1180 N. Federal Hwy.
Pompano Beach, FL 33062
(800) 327-3525
www.macksgrove.com

# SEEDS FOR GROWING HERBS AND VEGETABLES

Burpee
300 Park Avenue
Warminster, PA 18991
(800) 888-1447
www.burpee.com

Renee's Garden
7389 W. Zayante Road
Felton, CA 95018
(888) 880-7228
www.reneesgarden.com

Vermont Bean Seed Company
334 West Stroud Street
Randolph, WI 53956-1274
(800) 349-1071
www.vermontbean.com

Obviously if you are searching for the hard-to-find bean seed, you look for someone who specializes in beans. If it grows in the United States, Vermont Bean has it!

# VEGETARIAN FOODS

Boca Burger Company
www.bocafoods.com

Boca Burger, proven to be the best ready-made vegetarian burger on the market, is constantly increasing its product line. Many meat analogs contain added fat and sodium; however, Boca's Vegan Original Burger does not contain added fat or sodium. Be sure to read the ingredient lists of their other entrée offerings, as not all of them are no fat/no sodium. Go to www.bocafoods.com to find a retailer close to you.

# VIDALIA ONIONS

Bland Farms
PO Box 790
Alamo, TX 78516
(800) 843-2542
www.blandfarms.com

These unbelievably sweet onions are available only from May through July. However, Bland Farms sells other onion varieties and farm produce. Each order of onions (minimum ten pounds) comes with a free recipe booklet. Catalogs are available upon request.

# NUTRITIONAL ANALYSIS RESOURCES

Pennington, Jean A.T. *Bowes & Church's Food Values of Portions Commonly Used.* 17th ed. New York: Lippincott, 1998.

Pope, Jamie and Martin Katahn. www.fitday.com (a nutritional analysis website).

*T-Factor Fat Gram Counter.* New York: Norton, 1994.

# APPENDIX B
## Sources for Ongoing Support

Rice Diet Store
1644 Cole Mill Road
Durham, NC 27705
(919) 383-7276 ext. 221
www.ricedietstore.com

The Rice Diet Store has a wide selection of support tools for keeping a health journal (*Personal Journal for Health*, *T-Factor Fat Gram Counter*, and Progoff's *At a Journal Workshop*), enhancing daily activities (yoga DVDs, straps, and pedometers), and expanding meditation practices (Thich Nhat Hanh and Jon Kabat-Zinn CDs and books).

## SOURCES FOR MORE INFORMATION

### Best Newsletters Available to Support Less Than 20 percent Fat Nutritional Approaches or Vegetarian Lifestyles

Center for Science in the Public Interest
1875 Connecticut Avenue, N.W., Suite 300
Washington, DC 20009
(202) 332-9110
www.cspinet.org

Although this nutrition newsletter is not as ambitious with their sodium and fat recommendations as this book, it is the only newsletter that reports information consistently more progressive than the others on limiting fat and sodium. In addition to highlighting a practical comparative survey of some type of food each month, they also guide those interested in making a difference.

Vegetarian Dietetics
American Dietetic Association
120 S. Riverside Plaza, Suite 2000
Chicago, IL 60606
(800) 877-1600

*Vegetarian Dietetics* is a newsletter published by the Vegetarian Nutrition practice group of the American Dietetic Association. Although the publication is more interested in vegetarian diets, without particular concern for fat and salt intake, their "Review of Recent Literature" section is the best that I have read.

## Our Favorite Vegetarian Books

Despite their occasional lack of concern about sodium.

Ballentine, R. *Transition to Vegetarianism: An Evolutionary Step.* Honesdale, PA: The Himalayan International Institute, 1987.
———. *Diet and Nutrition: A Holistic Approach.* Honesdale, PA: The Himalayan International Institute, 1978.
Jamieson, Alex. *The Great American Detox Diet.* Rodale Press, 2005.
Any of Dr. John McDougall's books are highly recommended: http://www.drmcdougall.com. The recipes are basic and simple, as well as being very low in fat and sodium.
Any of Dr. Dean Ornish's books are also highly recommended. For

those seeking prevention and reversal of heart disease, his *Dr. Dean Ornish's Program for Reversing Heart Disease* (New York: Random House, 1990) is a must. *Eat More Weigh Less* (New York: HarperCollins, 2001) is Dr. Ornish's life choice program for losing weight safely while eating abundantly. Again, be mindful of sodium levels that may exceed your goals in some of the recipes.

Ornish, Dean, M.D. *Everyday Cooking with Dr. Dean Ornish*. Quill, 1996.

Robbins, J. *Diet for a New America*. Walpole, NH: Stillpoint Publishing, 1987. This is a tender, yet informative book on the health, humane, and political reasons for vegetarianism. Contains no recipes.

# Cookbooks with Low-Fat, Low-Sodium Recipes

American Heart Association. *Low Salt Cookbook*, 2nd ed. New York: Clarkson Potter, 2002.

Anderson, David C. *The No-Salt Cookbook*. Adams Media, 2001.

Bagg, Elma W. *Cooking Without a Grain of Salt*. New York: Bantam Books, 1998.

Gazzaniga, Donald. *The No-Salt, Lowest-Sodium Baking Book*. New York: St. Martin's Press, 2002.

Gittelman, Ann Louise, Ph.D., CNS. *Get the Salt Out*. New York: Three Rivers Press, 1996.

Mostyn, Bobbie. *Pocket Guide to Low Sodium Foods*. Indata, 1998.

Schell, M. *Chinese Salt-Free Diet Cookbook*. New York: New American Library.

Williams, J.B., and G. Silverman. *No Salt, No Sugar, No Fat Cookbook*. San Leandro, CA: Bristol Publishing Enterprises, 1982.

# Exemplary Nutrition

Hottinger, Greg. *The Best Natural Foods on the Market Today*, vol. 1. Boulder, CO: Huckleberry Mountain Press, 2004.

Schlosser, Eric. *Fast Food Nation: The Dark Side of the All-American Meal.* Houghton Mifflin, 2001.

Simopoulos, Artemis P., and Jo Robinson. *The Omega Diet: The Lifesaving Nutritional Program Based on the Diet of the Island of Crete.* New York: Harper Perennial, 1999.

# Books on Inner Healing

Brach, Tara. *Radical Acceptance: Embracing Your Life with the Heart of a Buddha.* New York: Bantam, 2003.

Bradshaw, John. *On: The Family.* Health Communications, Inc., 1996.

Bullitt-Jonas, Margaret. *Holy Hunger: A Woman's Journey from Food Addiction to Spiritual Fulfillment.* New York: Vintage Books, 2000.

Bushnell, Sheridan. *Stepping into the Circle: Healing Parables for a New Century.* Sonorous Press, 1998.

Damasio, Antonio. *Looking for Spinoza: Joy, Sorrow, and the Feeling Brain.* New York: Harcourt, 2003.

D'Arcy, Paula. *Seeking with All My Heart: Encountering God's Presence Today.* The Crossroad Carlisle Book, 2003.

Dyer, Wayne W. *There's A Spiritual Solution to Every Problem.* New York: HarperCollins, 2001.

Emoto, Masaru. *The Hidden Messages in Water.* Beyond Words Publishing, 2004.

Excerpts from *What the Bleep Do We Know!? The Little Book of BLEEPS.* Hillsboro, OR: Beyond Words, 2002.

Hendrix, Harville. *Getting the Love You Want: A Guide for Couples.* New York: HarperCollins, 1989.

Hoff, Benjamin. *The Tao of Pooh.* New York: Penguin Books, 1983.

Kabat-Zinn, Jon. *Full Catastrophe Living: Using the Wisdom of Your Body and Mind to Face Stress, Pain, and Illness.* New York: Dell, 1991. (In addition, relaxation and meditation tapes available from author.)

————. *Wherever You Go, There You Are: Mindfulness Meditation in Everyday Life.* New York: Hyperion, 1995.

Keating, Thomas. *Open Mind Open Heart: The Contemplative Dimension of the Gospel.* The Continuum Publishing Company, 1996.

Koenig, Harold G. *The Healing Power of Faith: Science Explores Medicine's Last Great Frontier.* New York: Simon & Schuster, 1999.

Kornfield, Jack. *A Path with Heart: A Guide through the Perils and Promises of Spiritual Life.* New York: Bantam Doubleday Dell Publishing Group, 1993.

Ledoux, Joseph. *The Emotional Brain: The Mysterious Underpinnings of Emotional Life.* New York: Simon & Schuster, 1998.

Lewis, Thomas, Fari Amini, and Richard Lannon. *A General Theory of Love.* New York: Vintage Books, 2001.

Miller, Alice. *The Drama of the Gifted Child: The Search for the True Self.* New York: HarperCollins, 1996.

Nhat Hahn, Thich: *Being Peace.* Parallax Press, 1988.

————. *Peace is Every Step.* New York: Bantam Books, 1991.

————. *The Blooming of a Lotus.* Beacon Press, 1993.

————. *The Miracle of Mindfulness: A Manual on Meditation.* Beacon Press, 1996.

————. *Teachings on Love.* Parallax Press, 1998.

————. *Anger: Wisdom for Cooling the Flames.* New York: Putnam, 2001.

————. *The Heart of the Buddha's Teaching: Transforming Suffering into Peace, Joy and Liberation.* Parallax Press, 1998.

Oriah Mountain Dreamer. *The Dance: Moving to the Rhythms of Your True Self.* San Francisco: Harper San Francisco, 2001.

Peck, M. Scott. *The Road Less Traveled: A New Psychology of Love,*

*Traditional Values and Spiritual Growth.* New York: Simon & Schuster, 1998.

———. *Golf and the Spirit: Lessons for the Journey.* New York: Random House, 1999.

Pert, Candace B. *Molecules of Emotion: The Science Behind Mind-Body Medicine.* New York: Simon & Schuster, 1997.

Progoff, Ira. *At a Journal Workshop: Writing to Access the Power of the Unconscious and Evoke Creative Ability.* Tarcher/Putnam, 1992.

Remen, Rachel Naomi. *Kitchen Table Wisdom: Stories That Heal.* Riverhead Books, 1996.

Robbins, John. *Diet for a New America.* Stillpoint, 1987. Reprint, Tilburon, CA: HJ Kramer; Novato, CA: New World Library, 1998.

Rubin, Lillian B. *Intimate Strangers: Men and Women Together.* New York: HarperCollins, 1984.

Ruiz, Don Miguel. *The Fouir Agreements: A Practical Guide to Personal Freedom.* Amber-Allen Publishing, 1997.

Salzberg, Susan. *Loving-Kindness: The Revolutionary Art of Happiness.* Boston: Shambhala Publications, 1995.

Siegel, Bernie. *Love, Medicine and Miracles: Lessons Learned About Self-Healing from a Surgeon's Experience with Exceptional Patients.* New York: Harper Perennial, 1990.

Wheelis, Allen. *How People Change.* New York: HarperCollins, 1974.

Whitfield, Charles L. *Healing the Child Within.* Health Communications, 1989.

*The 12 Steps.* The Oxford Group, RPI Publishing, 1995.
    *A Way Out*
    *A Spiritual Journey*

Weill, Andrew, M.D., *Spontaneous Healing: How to Discover and Embrace Your Body's Natural Ability to Maintain and Heal Itself.* New York: Ballantine, 2000.

———. *Eating Well For Optimum Health: The Essential Guide to Bringing Health and Pleasure Back to Eating.* New York: HarperCollins, 2001.

# Meditation Tapes and CDs

Jon Kabat-Zinn. *Mindfulness Meditation Practice Tapes.* May be obtained from Web site www.mindfulnesstapes.com, by mail from Stress Reduction Tapes, PO Box 547, Lexington, MA 02420, or from us.

Thich Nhat Hahn. *Plum Village Meditations: With Thich Nhat Hahn and Sister Jina Van Hengel.* Sounds True, 1997.

———. *Classic Dharma Talks.* Parallax Press.

*Looking Deeply: Mindfulness and Meditation.*

*Truly Seeing*

*Being Peace*

*Touching Peace*

# ANONYMOUS GROUPS

American Self Help Clearing House
100 E. Hanover Avenue, Suite 202
Cedar Knoll, NJ 07927-2020
(973) 326-6789
http://mentalhelp.net/selfhelp/

The Self-Help Sourcebook Online is a searchable database that includes information on more than 1,100 national-, international-, and demonstrational-model self-help support groups, ideas for starting groups, and opportunities to link with others to develop needed new national or international groups.

Hazelden Educational Materials
PO Box 11 CO3
Center City, MN 55012-0011
(800) 328-9000
Minnesota: (800) 257-0070
www.hazeldenbookplace.org

Hazelden Educational Materials publishes much of the 12-step Anonymous groups' literature.

Adult Children of Alcoholics (ACOA)
PO Box 3216
Torrance CA 90510
(310) 534-1815
www.adultchildren.org

ACOA groups do not require that you are literally a biological child of an alcoholic, but they are interested in examining your addictive behaviors, such as *controlling or enabling others*. ACOA and information on other anonymous groups may be found via a phone call to your local Alcoholics Anonymous (AA). As all the groups are different to some extent, try each group a few times before deciding which is best for you.

Overeaters Anonymous
World Service Office
PO Box 44020
Rio Rancho, NM 87174-4020
(505) 891-2664
www.oa.org

The website contains a locator that will assist you in locating a local chapter, or call your local AA.

# CENTERS FOR HEALING AND MEDITATION

Network for Attitudinal Healing International
33 Buchanan Street
Sausalito, CA 94965
(415) 331-6161
www.healingcenter.org

The Attitudinal Healing groups provide support for people who want to explore their abilities to perceive things differently, to choose peace rather than conflict, and love rather than fear. Groups are offered free with trained peer facilitators, on-line chat sites, and pay-to-attend conferences. For more call or click on the Web site.

The Legacy Center
2200 Gateway Centre Blvd., Suite 216
Morrisville, NC 27560
phone: (919) 678-6000
FAX: (919) 678-6015
www.TheLegacyCenter.com

The Legacy Center is a powerful experiential group program designed to assist those ready to actualize their life to the fullest. It leads you to realize the choice we all have to cocreate our life by "standing as source for a transformed world."

Green Mountain Dharma Center
(for women)
PO Box 182, Ayres Lane
Hartland-Four-Corners, VT 05049
phone: (802) 436-1103/1102
FAX: (802) 436-1101
e-mail: MF-office@plumvillage.org
www.greenmountaincenter.org

Deer Park Monastery
General Inquiry/Soldity Hamlet
(for men and couples)
2499 Melru Lane
Escondido, CA 92026
phone: (760) 291-1003
FAX: (760) 291-1010
e-mail: deerpark@plumvillage.org
www.deerparkmonastery.org

Maple Forest Monastery
(for men and couples)
PO Box 354
South Woodstock, VT 05071
phone: (802) 457-9442
FAX: (802) 457-8170
e-mail: stoneboy@vermontel.net
www.mapleforestmonastery.org

Deer Park Monastery
Clarity Hamlet
2499 Melru Lane
Escondido, CA 92026
phone: (760) 291-1029
FAX: (760) 291-1172
e-mail: clarity@plumvillage.org
www.deerparkmonastery.org

The above centers are all associated with Thich Nhat Hanh, who offers retreats and talks each summer in the United States. Also there are retreats year round at his retreat center, Plum Village, in France. For a schedule of retreats and other information, visit plumvillage.org or, in the United States, contact one of the retreat centers listed.

# CHRISTIAN RETREAT CENTERS

Aqueduct
716 Mount Carmel Church Road
Chapel Hill, NC 27514
(919) 933-5557

Aqueduct is an exceptional retreat center for emotional and spiritual healing nestled on a hill just south of Chapel Hill, North Carolina. Priests, preachers, or therapists who are especially gifted in healing conduct their retreats. They offer three-and-a-half-day retreats approximately monthly, complete with beautiful accommodations and a food service receptive to vegetarian requests.

Pecos Benedictine Monastery
Our Lady of Guadalupe Abbey
PO Box 1080
Pecos, NM 87552-1080
(505) 757-6415
www.pecosabbey.org

Snail's Pace
Attn: Melissa Lang
PO Box 593
633 Louisiana Ave
Saluda, NC 28773
(828) 749-3851

# APPENDIX C

## One-Day Food Intake Analysis

Try it and then see where you need to make adjustments.

| Portion and Food | Calories | Sodium (mg) | Fat (g) | SFA (g) | CHOL (mg) |
|---|---|---|---|---|---|
| **Breakfast:** | | | | | |
| _____ | ___ | ___ | ___ | ___ | ___ |
| _____ | ___ | ___ | ___ | ___ | ___ |
| _____ | ___ | ___ | ___ | ___ | ___ |
| _____ | ___ | ___ | ___ | ___ | ___ |
| **Lunch:** | | | | | |
| _____ | ___ | ___ | ___ | ___ | ___ |
| _____ | ___ | ___ | ___ | ___ | ___ |
| _____ | ___ | ___ | ___ | ___ | ___ |
| _____ | ___ | ___ | ___ | ___ | ___ |
| **Dinner:** | | | | | |
| _____ | ___ | ___ | ___ | ___ | ___ |
| _____ | ___ | ___ | ___ | ___ | ___ |
| _____ | ___ | ___ | ___ | ___ | ___ |
| _____ | ___ | ___ | ___ | ___ | ___ |
| **Totals for the day** | ☐ | ☐ | ☐ | ☐ | ☐ |
| **Rice Diet Guidelines →** | [1,000] | [500–1,000] | [22.2] | [5.5] | [0–100] |

1. Take total fat grams, multiply by 9, divide by total calories, and multiply by 100 to get percent of the day's intake coming from fat:

[(fat grams $\times$ 9)/total calories] $\times$ 100 = **% of intake from fat**

2. Take total saturated fat (SFA) grams, multiply by 9, divide by total calories, and multiply by 100 to get percent of the day's intake coming from saturated fat:

[(sat fat grams $\times$ 9)/total calories] $\times$ 100 = **% of intake from saturated fat**

# BIBLIOGRAPHY

## INTRODUCTION

Ard J.D., R.R., Oddone, E.Z. "Culturally-Sensitive Weight Loss Program Produces Significant Reduction in Weight, Blood Pressure, and Cholesterol in Eight Weeks." *Journal of the National Medical Association*, 2000. 92(11): pp. 515–23.

Kempner, W. "Some Effects of the Rice Diet Treatment of Kidney Disease and Hypertension." *Bull NY Acad Med*, 1946. 22: pp. 358–370.

———. "Treatment of Cardiac Failure with Rice Diet." *NC Med J*, 1947. 8: pp. 128–131.

———. "Treatment of Heart and Kidney Disease and of Hypertensive and Arteriosclerotic Vascular Disease with the Rice Diet. *Ann Int Med*, 1948. 31: pp. 687–688.

———. "Treatment of Hypertensive Vascular Disease with Rice Diet." *Am J Med*, 1948. 4: pp. 545–577.

———. "Treatment of Kidney Disease and Hypertensive Vascular Disease with Rice Diet." *NC Med J*, 1944. 5: pp. 125–133.

———. "Treatment of Kidney Disease and Hypertensive Vascular Disease with Rice Diet II." *NC Med J*, 1944. 5: pp. 273–274.

———. "Treatment of Kidney Disease and Hypertensive Vascular Disease with Rice Diet III." *NC Med J*, 1945. 6: pp. 61–87, 117–161.

———, N.B., Peschel, R.L., Skyler, J.S. "Treatment of Massive Obesity with Rice/Reduction Diet Program: An Analysis of 106 Patients with at Least a 45-Kg Weight Loss." *Archives of Internal Medicine*, 1975. 135(12): pp. 1575–84.

———. P.R., Schlayer, C. "Effects of Rice Diet on Diabetes Mellitus Associated with Vascular Disease." *Postgrad Med*, 1958. 24: pp. 359–371.


# CHAPTER ONE

Kempner, W. "Some Effects of the Rice Diet Treatment of Kidney Disease and Hypertension." *Bull NY Acad Med*, 1946. 22: pp. 358–370.

———. "Treatment of Cardiac Failure with Rice Diet." *NC Med J*, 1947. 8: pp. 128–131.

———. "Treatment of Heart and Kidney Disease and of Hypertensive and Arteriosclerotic Vascular Disease with the Rice Diet." *Ann Int Med*, 1948. 31: pp. 687–688.

———. "Treatment of Hypertensive Vascular Disease with Rice Diet." *Am J Med*, 1948. 4: pp. 545–577.

———. "Treatment of Kidney Disease and Hypertensive Vascular Disease with Rice Diet." Presented at *AMA*, Chicago: 1944.

———. "Treatment of Kidney Disease and Hypertensive Vascular Disease with Rice Diet." *NC Med J*, 1944. 5: pp. 125–133.

———. "Treatment of Kidney Disease and Hypertensive Vascular Disease with Rice Diet II." *NC Med J*, 1944. 5: pp. 273–274.

———. "Treatment of Kidney Disease and Hypertensive Vascular Disease with Rice Diet III." *NC Med J*, 1945. 6: pp. 61–87, 117–161.

———, N.B., Peschel, R.L., Skyler, J.S. "Treatment of Massive Obesity with Rice/Reduction Diet Program: An Analysis of 106 Patients with at Least a 45-Kg Weight Loss." *Archives of Internal Medicine*, 1975. 135(12): pp. 1575–84.

———, P.R., Schlayer, C. "Effects of Rice Diet on Diabetes Mellitus Associated with Vascular Disease." *Postgrad Med* 1958. 24: pp. 359–371.

Recovery, F.i., *The 12 Steps: A Spiritual Journey.* RPI Publishing, 1988, 1994.

Recovery, F.i., *The 12 Steps: A Way Out.* 1987, RPI Publishing, 1989, 1995.


# CHAPTER TWO

Hottinger, Greg M., R.D., *The Best Natural Foods on the Market Today.* Vol. 1. Boulder, CO: Huckleberry Mountain Press, 2004. pp. 187–188.


# CHAPTER FOUR

The American Cancer Society 1996 Advisory Committee on Diet, N., and Cancer Prevention. "Guidelines on Diet, Nutrition, and Cancer Prevention: Reducing the Risk of Cancer with Healthy Food Choices and Physical Activity." *CA Cancer J Clin.*, 1996. 46: pp. 325–341.

Anitschkow, N. "Experimental Arteriosclerosis in Animals." *Arteriosclerosis.* 1933 (In: Cowdry, E.V., ed.): pp. 271–322.

Armstrong, M., Warner, E.D., Connor, W.E. "Regression of Coronary Atheromatosis in Rhesus Monkeys." *Circ Res.*, 1970. 27: pp. 59–67.

Bank, F.D. *Nutritionist V Nutrition Software*, Version 2.3. 2000. San Bruno, CA: First Data Bank, 2000.

Burr, M.L., Gilbert, J.F., Deadman, N.M. "Effects of Changes in Fat, Fish, and Fibre Intakes on Death and Myocardial Reinfarction: Diet and Reinfarction Trial (DART)." *The Lancet*, 1989: pp. 757–761.

Connor, W. "Dietary Cholesterol and the Pathogenesis of Atherosclerosis." *Geriatrics*, 1961. 16: pp. 407–415.

Cordain, L., et al., "Origins and Evolution of the Western Diet: Health Implications for the 21st Century." *Am J Clin Nutr*, 2005. 81: pp. 341–354.

de Lorgeril, M., Renaud, S., Delaye, J. "Mediterranean Alpha-Linolenic Acid-Rich Diet in Secondary Prevention of Coronary Heart Disease. *The Lancet*, 1994. 343: pp. 1454–1455.

de Lorgeril, M., Salen, P., Delaye, J. "Effect of a Mediterranean Type of Diet on the Rate of Cardiovascular Complications in Patients with Coronary Artery Disease." *J Amer Coll Cardiology*, 1996. 28(5): pp. 1103–1108.

Dyerberg, J., Bband, H.O., Aagaard, O. " 'Small is beautiful': Alpha Linolenic Acid and Eicosapentaenoic Acid in Man." *The Lancet*, 1983: p. 1169.

Eaton, S.B. "An Evolutionary Perspective Enhances Understanding of Human Nutritional Requirements." *J Nutr*, 1996. 126: pp. 1732–1740.

Galloway, J. *The Cambridge World History of Food*. Vol. 1. Cambridge: Cambridge University Press, 2000.

Hottinger, G. *The Best Natural Foods on the Market Today*. Vol. 1. Boulder, CO: Huckleberry Mountain Press, 2004.

Jenkins, D., et al., "Glycemic Index of Foods: A Physiological Basis for Carbohydrate Exchange." *Am J Clin Nutr*, 1981. 34: pp. 362–366.

Kempner, K. "Compensation of Renal Metabolic Dysfunction." *NC Med J*, 1945. 6(2): pp. 61–87.

Kern, P.A, O.J., Saffari, B., Carty, J. "The Effects of Weight Loss on the Activity and Expression of Adipose-Tissue Lipoprotein Lipase in Very Obese Humans." *N Engl J Med*, 1990. 322: pp. 1053–1059.

Keys, A. *Seven Countries: A Multivariate Analysis of Death and Coronary Heart Disease*. Cambridge, MA: Harvard University Press, 1980.

Klem, M.L., et al. "Does Weight Loss Maintenance Become Easier Over Time?" *Obesity Research*, 2000. 8: pp. 438–444.

———, et al. "A Descriptive Study of Individuals Successful at Long-Term Maintenance of Substantial Weight Loss." *Am J Clin Nutrition*, 1997. 66: pp. 239–246.

Liu, S., Willett, W.C. "Dietary Glycemic Load and Atherothrombotic Risk." *Curr Atheroscler Rep*, 2002. 4: pp. 454–461.

McGuire, M.T., et al. "What Predicts Weight Regain Among a Group of Successful Weight Losers?" *J of Consulting and Clinical Psychology*, 1999. 67: pp. 177–185.

Nelson, J. "Wheat: Its Processing and Utilization." *Am J Clin Nutr*, 1985. 41: pp. 1070–1076.

Ornish, D., et al. "Can Lifestyle Changes Reverse Coronary Heart Disease?" *Lancet*, 1990. 336(1994): p. 129–133.

Pearce, M.L.a.S.D. "Incidence of Cancer in Men on a Diet High in Polyunsaturated Fat." *The Lancet*, 1971: pp. 464–467.

Reddy, S., et al., "Effect of Low Carbohydrate High-Protein Diets on Acid-Base Balance, Stone-Forming Propensity, and Calcium Metabolism." *Am J Kidney Dis.*, 2002. 40: p. 265–274.

Renaud, S., Paul, T. "Cretan Mediterranean Diet for Prevention of Coronary Heart Disease." *Am J Clin Nutr*, 1995. 61 (suppl): pp. 1360S–1367S.

Schlosser, E. *Fast Food Nation: The Dark Side of the All-American Meal.* New York: HarperPerennial, 2002.

Schuler, G., et al., "Myocardial Perfusion and Regression of Coronary Artery Disease in Patients on a Regimen of Intensive Physical Exercise and Low Fat Diet." *J. Amer College of Cardiology*, 1992. 19: pp. 34–42.

Simopoulos, A.P. "Omega-3 Fatty Acids in Health and Disease and in Growth and Development." *Am J Clin Nutr*, 1991. 54: pp. 438–463.

———. "The Role of Fatty Acids in Gene Expression: Health Implications." *Ann Nutr Metab*, 1996. 40: pp. 303–311.

———. *The Omega Diet: The Lifesaving Nutritional Program Based on the Diet of the Island of Crete.* New York: HarperPerennial, 1999.

Singh, J., Hamid, R., Reddy, B.S. "Dietary Fat and Colon Cancer: Modulating Effect of Types and Amount of Dietary Fat on Ras-p21 Function During Promotion and Progression Stages of Colon Cancer." *Cancer Research*, 1997. 57: pp. 253–258.

Storck, J. T.W. *Flour for Man's Bread, a History of Milling.* Minneapolis: University of Minnesota Press, 1952.

# CHAPTER FIVE

Kabat-Zinn, J. *Full Catastrophe Living: Using the Wisdom of Your Body and Mind to Face Stress, Pain, and Illness*. New York: Dell Publishing Company, 1991.

Nhat Hahn, Thich. *The Blooming of a Lotus*. Beacon Press, 1993.

# CHAPTER SEVEN

Jampolsky, G. *Love is Letting Go of Fear*, revised ed. San Francisco: Celestial Arts; 1988.

Koenig, H. "Religion, Spirituality and Medicine: Research Findings and Implications for Clinical Practice." *Southern Med Journal*, 2004. 97: pp. 1194–1200.

Koenig, H.G., M.D. *The Healing Connection*. Philadelphia: Templeton Foundation Press, 2004.

———. *The Healing Power of Faith*. New York: Simon & Schuster, 2001.

———. Larson, D.B. *The Handbook of Religion and Health*. New York: Oxford University Press, 2001.

# CHAPTER EIGHT

Bjelakovic, G. et al., "Antioxidant Supplements for Prevention of Gastrointestinal Cancers: A Systematic Review and Meta-Analysis." *Lancet*, 2004. 364: pp. 1219–1228.

Egan, B., "Biochemical and Metabolic Effects of Very-Low-Salt Diets." *Am J Med Science*, 2000. 320(4): pp. 233–239.

Group, H.P.S.C., "MRC/BHF Heart Protection Study of Antioxidant

Vitamin Supplementation in 20 536 High-Risk Individuals: A Randomised Placebo-Controlled Trial." *Lancet*, 2002. 360: pp. 23–33.

Kempner, W. "Some Effects of the Rice Diet Treatment of Kidney Disease and Hypertension." *Bull NY Acad Med*, 1946. 22: pp. 358–370.

———. "Treatment of Cardiac Failure with Rice Diet." *NC Med J*, 1947. 8: pp. 128–131.

———. "Treatment of Heart and Kidney Disease and of Hypertensive and Arteriosclerotic Vascular Disease with the Rice Diet." *Ann Int Med*, 1948. 31: pp. 687–688.

———. "Treatment of Hypertensive Vascular Disease with Rice Diet." *Am J Med*, 1948. 4: pp. 545–577.

———. "Treatment of Kidney Disease and Hypertensive Vascular Disease with Rice Diet." *NC Med J*, 1944. 5: pp. 125–133.

———. "Treatment of Kidney Disease and Hypertensive Vascular Disease with Rice Diet II." *NC Med J*, 1944. 5: pp. 273–274.

———. "Treatment of Kidney Disease and Hypertensive Vascular Disease with Rice Diet III." *NC Med J*, 1945. 6: pp. 61–87, 117–161.

———, N.B., Peschel, R.L., Skyler, J.S. "Treatment of Massive Obesity with Rice/Reduction Diet Program: An Analysis of 106 Patients with at Least a 45-Kg Weight Loss." *Archives of Internal Medicine*, 1975. 135(12): pp. 1575–1584.

———, P.R., Schlayer, C. "Effects of Rice Diet on Diabetes Mellitus Associated with Vascular Disease." *Postgrad Med* 1958. 24: pp. 359–371.

Ornish, D., et al., "Can Lifestyle Changes Reverse Coronary Heart Disease?" *Lancet*, 1990. 336: pp. 129–133.

Rosati, K.G. *Heal Your Heart: The New Rice Diet Program for Reversing Heart Disease Through Nutrition, Exercise and Spiritual Renewal.* New York: Wiley & Sons, 1997.

Sellmeyer, D. et al, "A High Ratio of Dietary Animal to Vegetable Protein Increases the Rate of Bone Loss and the Risk of Fracture in Postmenopausal Women." *AJCN*, 2001. 73(1): pp. 118–122.

Thorburn, A. "Salt and the Glycaemic Response." *British Medical Journal*, 1986. 292: pp. 1697–1699.

# FINAL NOTE

C.L. Distribution, *The Little Book of Bleeps: Quotations from the Movie . . . What the Bleep Do We Know!?* Hillsboro, OR: Beyond Words, 2005.

# ACKNOWLEDGMENTS

A special thank you and lots of love and gratitude go to everyone who has committed to the Rice Diet Program and to the dream of extending this healing message to many, many more people. It has been a long-held dream to have our phenomenal history and healing potential shared with those who are ready to reclaim their lives and health. So many have contributed to this book, from participants with personal success stories quoted within to many others whose courageous example and unspoken commitments to healing themselves naturally inspire others to do likewise. These undiscovered stars shine brightly here as they pass their torch on to others by standing steadfast to their commitment to maximize their lives.

This book was divinely timed. Our editor, Amanda Murray, called it forth after reading a *New York Times* front-page article highlighting the Rice Diet Program's weight loss history and success, and within two weeks more miracles happened faster than any of us had ever witnessed in our publishing experience. It has truly been a healing of my previously held "scarcity of time" belief system. I now believe that anything can happen in less time than any of us can imagine. Thank you Amanda, Debra Goldstein (our agent), and Billie Fitzpatrick (our collaborator). I'm not sure which is more powerful: a truth whose time has come, or four women with the same intention and commitment! All we really know is to praise God from whom all blessings flow.

The many who have contributed are really too numerous to thank here. Thank you, Dr. Kempner and all the early visionaries who had the courage to empower their patients to take responsibility for their health, promoting dietary choices. And, more currently, the incredible staff that supports and encourages our participants and us daily, and with this book's birthing specifically. Blessings on you, Dr. Neelon, Rachelle Fong, Susan Levy, Jayne Charles, Jeff Georgi, Judy Rivers (since June 15, 1964), Betsy Hamilton, Chef J.R., Nancy, Beverly, Ms. Betty (since February 27, 1967), and Ken Rosati. Our Rice Diet family also includes the loving instruction and support from Joy Anandi, Dr. Jay Dunbar, Dr. Eilene Bisgrove, Dr. Harold Koenig, Dr. Siegfried Heyden, Patricia Esperon, Ronnie Kolotkin, Di Di Dutrow, Helene Mau, Kathy Bryson, Pat Carlson, Helen Moran, Susan Hunnings, Adele Truslow, Jan Croft, and Karen Winstead. The divine timing was evident for this book's timely birth even in the way interns came to us with the gifts needed to finish the job. Thank you, Heidi Chen, Parker Freeman, and Kym Stork, whose contributions were completed just in time, teaching me again that we have all the time we need if we are standing as source for a transformed world. And thanks to Legacy, a leadership training program, that has recently inspired me to a deeper level of "sourcing," or "cocreating" my dreams and intentions.

# GENERAL INDEX

# RECIPE INDEX